COLOR ATLAS AND SYNOPSIS OF SEXUALLY TRANSMITTED DISEASES

COLOR ATLAS AND SYNOPSIS OF SEXUALLY TRANSMITTED DISEASES

SECOND EDITION

H. Hunter Handsfield, M.D.

Professor of Medicine
University of Washington School of Medicine
Director, STD Control Program
Department of Public Health – Seattle & King County
Seattle, Washington

McGraw-Hill
MEDICAL PUBLISHING DIVISION

New York   St. Louis   San Francisco   Auckland   Bogotá   Caracas   Lisbon
London   Madrid   Mexico City   Milan   Montreal   New Delhi
San Juan   Singapore   Sydney   Tokyo   Toronto

McGraw-Hill

A Division of The **McGraw·Hill** Companies

COLOR ATLAS AND SYNOPSIS OF SEXUALLY TRANSMITTED DISEASES,
Second Edition

Copyright © 2001, 1991 by *The **McGraw-Hill** Companies, Inc.* All rights
reserved. Printed in the United States of America. Except as permitted under
the United States Copyright Act of 1976, no part of this publication may be
reproduced or distributed in any form or by any means, or stored in a data
base or retrieval system, without prior written permission of the publisher.

1234567890 KGPKGP 09876543210

ISBN 0-07-026033-8

This book was set in Times Roman by York Graphic Services
The editors were Martin Wonsiewicz, Kathleen McCullough, and Scott Kurtz
The production supervisor was Richard Ruzycka.
The cover designer was Mary Skudlarek.
The index was prepared by Edwin Durbin.
Quebecor World/Kingsport was printer and binder.

This book is printed on acid-free paper.

Library of Congress Cataloging in Publication Data

Handsfield, H. Hunter.
    Color atlas and synopsis of sexually transmitted diseases / author, H. Hunter
Handsfield.—2nd ed.
        p. ; cm.
    Includes bibliographical references and index.
    ISBN 0-07-026033-8
        1. Sexually transmitted diseases—Atlases. 2. Sexually transmitted diseases—Outlines,
syllabi, etc. I. Title.
    [DNLM: 1. Sexually Transmitted Diseases—Atlases. WC 17 H236c 2001]
    RC200 .H36 2001
    616.95′1—dc21

                                                                              00-041552

For Patricia, Lara, Evan, and Kate

CONTENTS

Section V Clinical Syndromes   **137**

Until fifty years ago, venereal diseases were part of the medical mainstream, but following the development of penicillin—widely believed to herald the end of the "venereal disease problem" as well as other infectious diseases—venereology became a backwater field, and clinical care for "that kind" of patient was relegated to underfunded, poorly equipped clinics staffed by undertrained and often unenthusiastic clinicians. Thus, the medical professions and public health systems were unprepared for three developments. First, demographic and social changes—the sexual revolution, the worldwide population explosion, and global urbanization and population migration—placed most people at risk for sexually transmitted diseases for much of their lives. STDs never had been limited to "that kind" of patient, but now it became obvious. Second, advances in microbiology, immunology, and epidemiology defined a panoply of previously unrecognized STDs, many of which were difficult to recognize and hard to treat, yet caused serious, long-lasting sequelae. The third development was the explosive appearance of AIDS, the most devastating STD of all time.

STDs are among the most common afflictions in all societies. At least one half of the U.S. population acquires one or more sexually transmitted infections; indeed, genital human papillomavirus alone probably infects over half of all sexually active persons, and at least a quarter of the population has genital herpes simplex virus infections. STDs are the most common antecedents of ectopic pregnancy and tubal infertility in women, and the sexually transmitted nature of cervical cancer, still one of the most common malignancies in women, is underappreciated by the public and clinicians alike. In addition to the "new" STDs such as chlamydial infection, genital herpes, and human papillomavirus infection, the traditional ones, especially syphilis and gonorrhea, continue to pose serious health problems; the classic STDs are causing tremendous havoc in most developing countries and the newly liberated states of Eastern Europe. Finally there is AIDS—a disease that is spread with special efficiency in the presence of other STDs, an exceedingly vicious circle.

Nevertheless, most health care providers and health sciences students receive little education about STDs other than AIDS, and in industrialized countries most complete their training with little or no hands-on experience in STD diagnosis and management. This atlas and synopsis is designed as a quick ride up the learning curve for clinicians who find themselves—sometimes to their surprise—caring for patients with STD or at risk and who need an easy-to-use aid to diagnosis and management. All the clinical and diagnostic procedures described in this book are well within the capability of the basically trained clinician, and most of the necessary laboratory tests are readily available at reasonable cost. This book also can be a visual aid in counseling patients and others at risk for STD. Health educators, public health administrators, and many persons in the general population will find it useful as well.

The case histories presented in this book are real, although some are composites of more than one patient. For some cases that occurred several years ago, the treatments described or tests performed have been updated to conform with current recommendations. Most of the photographs were taken of the patients described in the case summaries, but some were matched with other patients whose histories were known. Although the clinical photos will assist greatly in recognition of STDs, the synopses that begin each chapter can stand on their own. Indeed, the chapters on some STDs with manifestations that are not readily visualized except by invasive procedures have fewer photographs; one chapter has no photos at all. About one third of the clinical photographs are new for the second edition, and the synopses were completely rewritten to reflect updated epidemiology, treatment recommendations, and other developments.

As with most books, this one would not have been possible without the generous assistance of many colleagues. Rick Berger, Karl Beutner, Fred Bushnell, Connie Celum, Ann Collier, Larry Corey, John Douglas, David Eschenbach, Gavin Hart, Sharon Hillier, King Holmes, Mac Hooton, Phil Kirby, Barbara Krekeler, John Krieger, Sheila Lukehart, Jeanne Marrazzo, Steve Medwell, David Soper, Pål Wølner-Hanssen, David Spach, Walter Stamm, Claire Stevens, Christina Surawicz, Anna Wald, Wil Whittington, Bob Willkens, and Bob Wood loaned photographs, reviewed chapters, or otherwise provided assistance with this edition, the first one, or both. The staff of the Public Health – Seattle & King County Sexually Transmitted Disease Clinic referred many patients for photography, and their probing questions have kept me on my toes. I took many of the clinical photographs; others were taken by Roger Hartley of Pan Enterprises. Those loaned by colleagues or previously published elsewhere are credited, but the provenance of some slides in my collection is uncertain; I apologize to the owners if some were not appropriately credited. Thanks as well to Kitty McCullough, developmental editor. Finally, Marty Wonsiewicz, my publisher, deserves special thanks for his understanding, tact, and patience with my tardiness in preparing this edition.

Finally, I thank my wife, Patricia McInturff, for prodding me to complete both editions and tolerating the resulting erosion of our personal time.

H. Hunter Handsfield
Seattle, Washington
August 3, 2000

AGUS	atypical glandular cells of undetermined significance
AIDS	acquired immunodeficiency syndrome
ALT	alanine aminotransferase
ASCUS	atypical squamous cells of undetermined significance
bid	twice a day
BV	bacterial vaginosis
CDC	Centers for Disease Control and Prevention
CLIA	Clinical Laboratory Improvement Act
CMV	cytomegalovirus
CNS	central nervous system
CSF	cerebrospinal fluid
DGI	disseminated gonococcal infection
DNA	deoxyribonucleic acid
ESR	erythrocyte sedimentation rate
FTA-ABS	fluorescent treponemal antibody-absorbed test
HAV	hepatitis A virus
HBV	hepatitis B virus
HCV	hepatitis C virus
HDV	hepatitis D virus
HIV	human immunodeficiency virus
HLA	histocompatibility locus A
HPV	human papillomavirus
HSIL	high-grade squamous intraepithelial lesions
HSV	herpes simplex virus
ICGND	intracellular gram-negative diplococci
IDU	injection drug use/user
IM	intramuscularly
IV	intravenously
KSV	Kaposi's sarcoma virus
LCR	ligase chain reaction
LGV	lymphogranuloma venereum
LSIL	low-grade squamous intraepithelial lesions
MAC	*Mycobacterium avium* complex
MCV	Molluscum contagiosum virus
MHA-TP	microhemagglutination assay for *Treponema pallidum*
MPC	mucopurulent cervicitis
MSM	men who have sex with men
NGU	nongonococcal urethritis
PCR	polymerase chain reaction
PEP	post-exposure prophylaxis
PID	pelvic inflammatory disease
PMN	polymorphonuclear leukocyte
PO	orally, by mouth
PRN	as needed
qid	four times a day
RIBA	radioimmunoblot assay
RNA	ribonucleic acid
RPR	rapid plasma reagin test
STD	sexually transmitted disease
tid	three times a day
TMA	transcription-mediated amplification
TPPA	*Treponema pallidum* particle agglutination test
UTI	urinary tract infection
VDRL	Venereal Disease Research Laboratory test
VIN	vulvar intraepithelial neoplasia
VVC	vulvovaginal candidiasis
WSW	women who have sex with women

REVISED STD TREATMENT GUIDELINES

Shortly after this book went to press, the Centers for Disease Control and Prevention (CDC) convened a meeting of experts to consider revisions of CDC's recommendations for STD treatment. Although many of the modifications were anticipated in this book, clinicians are encouraged to consult the *2001 Guidelines for Treatment of Sexually Transmitted Diseases*, scheduled for publication in the spring of 2001, for possible changes in some of the recommended approaches. Likely modifications include:

- Endorsement of levofloxacin 250 mg orally as an option for initial single-dose therapy of uncomplicated gonorrhea.
- Consideration of ceftriaxone as an option for treatment of penicillin-allergic patients with infectious syphilis or neurosyphilis.
- Azithromycin is likely to be recommended for syphilis in doses of 1.0 g orally as postexposure prophylaxis and 2.0 g orally (or twice, one week apart) as treatment for primary or secondary syphilis, only when penicillin is contraindicated or injection therapy is not practical, and the patient is unlikely to adhere to multiple-dose therapy with doxycycline.
- Addition of levofloxacin, meropenem, and other drugs as options for the treatment of pelvic inflammatory disease.
- Addition of valacyclovir 500 mg twice daily for only 3 days as an option for episodic treatment of recurrent genital herpes.
- Recommendation of topical permethrin as the treatment of choice for pregnant women with scabies, and deletion of sulfur in petrolatum as a recommended regimen.

Other new treatments may be recommended, and the revised guidelines will include modified approaches to screening, diagnosis, counseling, partner management, and other prevention strategies for some STDs.

COLOR ATLAS AND SYNOPSIS OF SEXUALLY TRANSMITTED DISEASES

OVERVIEW OF SEXUALLY TRANSMITTED DISEASES

Chapter 1
CLINICAL APPROACH TO PATIENTS WITH STDs OR AT RISK

INTRODUCTION

In few areas of infectious diseases have changes in epidemiology and our understanding of clinical manifestations been as profound as in the field of sexually transmitted diseases (STDs) during the past three decades. Although the bacterial STDs declined in the 1990s in the United States and Western Europe, they remain epidemic in much of the world and in many parts of this country. Indeed, the United States has many times higher rates of the classic bacterial STDs than any other industrialized country, demonstrating the influence of demographic, social, and behavioral factors on infectious diseases despite availability of effective diagnosis and treatment. Sexually transmitted diseases embody all the elements of "emerging" infections, including recognition of new or apparently new pathogens, syndromes and complications, emergence of antimicrobial resistance in formerly susceptible pathogens, the increasing importance of viral infections, and rapid international spread fostered by the revolution in international travel and commerce.

Prevention and control of STDs are largely women's health care issues. Many STDs appear to be transmitted more efficiently from men to women than the reverse, probably because the exposed surface area is larger in women, the vagina serves as a reservoir that prolongs exposure to infectious secretions, and the risk of microscopic or overt traumatic injuries during intercourse may be greater in women than in men. Women are more likely than men to have subclinical or entirely asymptomatic infections, and the diagnosis of STD is more difficult in women because the clinical findings are less specific and some microbiologic tests are less sensitive in detecting disease in women than in men. Most important, women and their children are at much greater risk than men for long-lasting or permanent sequelae. Unfortunately, most STDs other than acquired immunodeficiency syndrome are considered minor conditions that do not justify the utilization of public resources for prevention.

Most persons are at substantial risk for STD during their teen and young adult years. More than 20 percent of the U.S. population acquires genital herpes simplex virus type 2 (HSV-2) infection by age 40; more than half of all women acquire genital human papillomavirus (HPV) infection within their first three or four lifetime sex partners; and each year 5 million and 3 million persons are estimated to acquire trichomoniasis and genital *Chlamydia trachomatis* infection, respectively. It is likely that well over one half of all Americans acquire one or more STDs sometime in their lives, and complications continue to occur for years after adoption of lower risk lifestyles. Virtually all primary care clinicians and many specialists regularly provide care to patients with STDs or their sequelae. As for all medical conditions, clinical recognition and diagnosis are central to treatment and prevention, and these are the focus of this book. This chapter presents an overview of the clinical approach to STD diagnosis and management.

CLASSIFICATION OF STDS

Sexually transmitted diseases can be classified according to the causative pathogens (see Table 1–1). However, many STD syndromes are caused by more than one STD pathogen, and in some cases nonsexually transmitted agents contribute to pathogenesis. Table 1–2 lists the major STD clinical syndromes and sequelae in order of their public health importance. (Note that the first half of Table 1–2 is dominated by syndromes that predominantly affect women and children.) Both the etiologic and syndromic organizations are used in this book.

Table 1–1 SEXUALLY TRANSMITTED PATHOGENS

Bacteria	Viruses
Neisseria gonorrhoeae	Human immunodeficiency virus (types 1 and 2)
Treponema pallidum	Herpes simplex virus (types 1 and 2)
Chlamydia trachomatis	Human papillomavirus (many types)
Haemophilus ducreyi	Hepatitis viruses A, B, C, and D
Calymmatobacterium granulomatis	Cytomegalovirus
Ureaplasma urealyticum	Epstein-Barr virus
Mycoplasma hominis	Molluscum contagiosum virus
Mycoplasma genitalium	Enteric viruses
Gardnerella vaginalis	
Salmonella species	
Shigella species	
Campylobacter species	
Streptococcus group B	
Mobiluncus species	

Protozoa	Ectoparasites
Trichomonas vaginalis	*Phthirus pubis* (pubic louse)
Entamoeba histolytica	*Sarcoptes scabiei* (scabies mite)
Giardia lamblia	
Other enteric protozoa	

Table 1–2 MAJOR STD CLINICAL SYNDROMES AND COMPLICATIONS

1. Acquired immunodeficiency syndrome and related conditions
2. Pelvic inflammatory disease
3. Female infertility and ectopic pregnancy
4. Fetal and neonatal infections: conjunctivitis, pneumonia, pharyngeal infection, encephalitis, cognitive impairment, deformities, deafness, immunodeficiency, death
5. Complications of pregnancy and delivery: spontaneous abortion, premature labor, premature rupture of fetal membranes, chorioamnionitis, postpartum endometritis
6. Neoplasia: cervical dysplasia and carcinoma, Kaposi's sarcoma, hepatocellular carcinoma, squamous cell carcinomas of anus, vulva, and penis
7. Human papillomavirus infection and genital warts
8. Genital ulcer–inguinal lymphadenopathy syndromes
9. Lower genital tract infection in women: cervicitis, urethritis, vaginal infection
10. Viral hepatitis and cirrhosis
11. Urethritis in men
12. Late syphilis
13. Epididymitis
14. Gastrointestinal infections: proctitis, enteritis, colitis
15. Acute arthritis
16. Mononucleosis syndrome
17. Molluscum contagiosum
18. Ectoparasite infestation (scabies, pubic lice)

POPULATIONS AT RISK

Recognition of the social and demographic markers for STD is the first step in assessing risk and in clinical management. Population subgroups with the frequencies of new sexual partnerships and other behavioral factors that sustain an STD in the community are defined as "core transmitters," sometimes called "spread clusters." Other persons acquire STD by sexual contact with core transmitters, but infection is not indefinitely propagated outside the core.

A primary determinant of core transmission is the mean duration of infection in the population. Gonorrhea, syphilis, and chancroid, for example, are transmissible only for days to weeks because therapeutic intervention and spontaneous resolution limit most cases, so that propagation of infection depends on infected persons having new sex partners within a brief interval after acquisition. Genital herpes and herpes simplex virus (HPV) infection, however, persist and are transmissible for many months or years, so that low rates of partner change—rates that are typical throughout society—are sufficient to sustain transmission. Therefore, the classic bacterial STDs are seen primarily in small subsets of the population that have high rates of partner change, which are often characterized by poverty, substance abuse, and prejudice, whereas the chronic viral STDs are common in all segments of society, including persons apparently at low risk. Chlamydial infection is intermediate: infection usually is more prolonged than gonorrhea but less so than HSV or HPV infection, so that chlamydial infection is seen in a broader segment of the population than gonorrhea but is less widespread than the viral STDs. Although the term *core group* is usually applied to young, ethnic minority persons of low socioeconomic level who have high rates of illicit drug use and prostitution, technically these are characteristics only of the core transmitters of the classic bacterial STDs. The core group for chlamydial infection probably is composed of most sexually active young persons, and that for genital herpes and HPV is most of the population.

STDs AND SEXUAL ORIENTATION

In the United States and most industrialized countries, men who have sex with men (MSM)—gay and bisexual men, plus others who may not acknowledge homosexual or bisexual orientation—had extraordinarily high rates of STDs in the 1970s and early 1980s. Rates of gonorrhea, syphilis, and enteric infections in MSM then declined rapidly as a result of behavioral changes in response to the appearance of AIDS. However, reported STD rates in MSM remained substantially higher than those in most exclusively heterosexual populations. In the late 1990s, STD rates began to climb yet again in MSM in cities throughout the United States, perhaps because dramatic advances in human immunodeficiency virus (HIV) therapy and survival led to lessened concern about AIDS. The situation is particularly explosive because more than half the MSM with syphilis in Seattle in 1998 and 20% of those with gonorrhea or chlamydial infection also were infected with HIV, and many acquired their infections in bath houses and other venues where unsafe sex with anonymous partners is especially common. Because most partners were anonymous, traditional partner notification was not effective as a control measure. Clinicians who provide care to MSM, both with and without HIV infection, should not assume that their patients have continued to follow safer sex guidelines; periodic STD screening and counseling are indicated for many such persons.

In contrast with MSM and exclusively heterosexual persons, lesbians and other women who have sex with women (WSW) apparently have relatively low rates of the classical STDs. Some STDs, such as genital HPV infection, and sexually associated diseases, such as bacterial vaginosis, are, however, common in WSW, including those who do not have sex with men. Clinicians should be alert to the possibility of STDs in WSW, including those who are exclusively lesbian.

INTERACTIONS BETWEEN HIV INFECTION AND OTHER STDS

Human immunodeficiency virus (HIV) infection is the most devastating STD of all time, far exceeding the morbidity and social impact of syphilis in the pre–antibiotic era. Moreover, HIV interacts with other STDs biologically, and behavioral and social factors further contribute to the transmission of HIV. Perhaps most important, the presence of inflammatory STDs markedly enhances the efficiency with which HIV is transmitted or acquired during sexual exposure. Genital herpes, syphilis, chancroid, gonorrhea, chlamydial infection, and trichomoniasis all have been shown in both cross-sectional and cohort studies to increase the likelihood of HIV transmission or acquisition 2-fold to as much as 32-fold. In HIV-infected persons, many of the inflammatory cells recruited to infected mucosal surfaces or ulcers are producing HIV in large numbers, and in those without HIV infection the same cells are especially susceptible to the virus if exposed. On a population basis, the prevalence of traditional STDs strongly predicts the likelihood and frequency of heterosexual transmission of HIV; indeed, the background prevalence and incidence of STDs may be the main explanation for differences in the frequency of heterosexually transmitted HIV around the world and between populations within countries. Thus, STD prevention is a crucial HIV prevention strategy.

In addition, STDs may adversely affect the clinical course of HIV disease, and vice versa. For example, among HIV-infected persons with recurrent genital herpes, HSV reactivation is accompanied by a substantial rise in plasma HIV viral load, perhaps affecting the progression of immunodeficiency. Compared with HIV-uninfected persons, those with HIV have more prolonged, painful, and debilitating HSV infections and a higher incidence of infection with acyclovir-resistant HSV strains; higher rates of antibiotic treatment failure for syphilis and chancroid; more rapid progression of genital or anal HPV infection to cancer or premalignant cellular changes; and perhaps higher frequencies and severity of pelvic inflammatory disease.

STD HISTORY AND PHYSICAL EXAMINATION

Assessment of STD risk requires an accurate social and sexual history, including appraisal of factors that influence sexuality, such as substance abuse. Broaching these subjects may be daunting, because the clinician may have personal anxieties and perceptions or may lack specific training about sexuality and, perhaps most important, because the process is viewed as requiring more time than a busy practice may allow. However, a forthright and sensitive approach usually elicits accurate information and often takes only 2 or 3 min. The medical history also can be succinct, yet complete.

The physical examination of patients with STD or at risk also is straightforward. In the author's STD clinic, we inspect all skin surfaces that are normally exposed during a genital examination, including the face, head, hands, lower arms, lower trunk, pubic area, buttocks, and thighs. The mouth and throat are examined, and the neck, supraclavicular fossae, axillae, and inguinal areas are palpated for lymphadenopathy. In men, the genitals and the pubic and inguinal regions are carefully inspected; the penis is palpated, including "milking" the urethra to assess for urethral discharge; and the scrotal contents are palpated for masses, tenderness, and other abnormalities. For homosexually active men, the anus and perineum are carefully inspected. The examination of women includes meticulous inspection of the external genitals, perineum, and anus; speculum examination of the vaginal mucosa and cervix; and a bimanual pelvic examination. For men or women with symptoms suggestive of proctitis or with lesions of the anus, the rectal mucosa is examined through an anoscope. The Appendix presents the elements of the medical and sexual history and the physical examination routinely conducted in the author's STD clinic.

LABORATORY DIAGNOSIS

Clinicians who manage patients with STD or at risk should have immediate access to serological tests for HIV infection and syphilis, type-specific HSV antibody tests, and specific tests for *Neisseria gonorrhoeae, Chlamydia trachomatis,* and HSV in genital secretions or ulcers. Although regulations resulting from the Clinical Laboratory Improvement Act (CLIA) have made office-based microscopy problematical in some settings, it is desirable to have immediate access to Gram-stained smears and wet mounts of vaginal secretions. Darkfield microscopy and rapid, point-of-service serological tests for syphilis should be available in offices and clinics that serve patient populations with high rates of syphilis.

- Most cases of *C. trachomatis* infection will not be detected without laboratory testing because clinical diagnosis and the epidemiologic predictors of infection are insensitive and nonspecific. The nucleic acid amplification assays, polymerase chain reaction (PCR), ligase chain reaction (LCR), and transcription-mediated amplification (TMA) are the tests of choice; their sensitivities are 90–95%, compared with only 60–70% for the antigen-detection or nonamplified DNA probe tests and 70–80% for isolation in tissue culture. The amplification tests also have the advantage of retaining excellent sensitivity on self-obtained vaginal swabs and on urine in both men and women, permitting testing in settings where collecting a urethral or cervical specimen is impractical.

- All cases of gonorrhea should be confirmed by specific laboratory tests. Isolation of the organism is increasingly being supplanted by antigen-detection or nonamplified DNA probe tests, or by DNA amplification methods, such as LCR and PCR. Unlike the chlamydia tests, however, culture remains highly sensitive and inexpensive and has the advantage of preserving isolates for antimicrobial susceptibility testing.
- Classic cases of genital herpes often can be diagnosed by history and physical examination, but atypical or nonspecific-appearing genital ulcers are the most common clinical manifestation. Herpes is by far the most frequent cause of genital ulceration, even in populations selected because of high rates of syphilis or chancroid. Tests to detect HSV are, therefore, indicated for all sexually active patients with genital ulcer disease. Isolation of the virus by tissue culture is the test of choice, but PCR assays are more sensitive and may be commercially available in the future. Type-specific serological assays, which accurately distinguish herpes simplex virus type 2 (HSV-2) from HSV type 1 (HSV-1) antibody, are indicated for many patients with genital ulcer disease, the sex partners of persons with genital herpes, and perhaps for screening. Until recently, most assays claiming to be type-specific did not accurately distinguish HSV-1 from HSV-2 infection; those older assays should be used rarely, if ever, for STD diagnosis.
- Serological tests for HIV should be routinely offered to most persons with STD or those at risk. Serological tests for syphilis continue to be indicated for those living in geographic areas known to have numerous cases of HIV and for populations in which syphilis persists in significant numbers. In some settings, serological tests for past or current hepatitis virus (A, B, or C) infection should be employed.
- The most common causes of vaginal discharge in young women—bacterial vaginosis, trichomoniasis, candidiasis, and mucopurulent cervicitis—often are difficult to differentiate clinically, and require microscopic or microbiologic tests. Rapid, point-of-service tests for semiquantitation of *Gardnerella vaginalis* or other rapid test methods may supplant microscopic examination of wet mount for the diagnosis of bacterial vaginosis in some settings. Although microscopy detects most cases of trichomoniasis or candidiasis, cultures for *Trichomonas vaginalis* and vaginal yeasts are underutilized.
- Papanicolaou (Pap) smears should be routinely obtained in women with STD or at risk, because they have the highest prevalences of premalignant dysplasia and overt malignancy. The role of tests for HPV infection in routine cervical cytology is, however, controversial; ongoing research should help to clarify this issue in the future. Anal pap smears often reveal premalignant dysplasia in MSM, especially in HIV-infected men. However, the role of routine anal cytology is not yet certain.

PRINCIPLES OF STD TREATMENT

Although *etiologic* treatment, therapy directed toward a documented pathogen, is often considered the ideal approach, most patients with STDs are treated presumptively. For example, most chlamydial infections in men are treated when they present with nongonococcal urethritis (NGU), whether or not attempts are made to document *C. trachomatis*. Similarly, to maximize therapeutic effectiveness, prevent complications, and prevent transmission to additional sex partners, most patients with genital herpes, syphilis, and other STDs are treated presumptively. True etiologic treatment is most commonly employed in screening programs in which infections are diagnosed in the absence of symptoms or signs.

Syndromic management is presumptive diagnosis and therapy made on the basis of standardized clinical and epidemiologic criteria; the term usually implies that no attempt will be made to document infection by specific laboratory tests. Promoted primarily for use in developing countries, syndromic treatment has a limited role in STD management in the United States.

Directly observed single-dose treatment has a special role in STD management. This strategy preceded the emergence of directly observed therapy as a mainstay of the tuberculosis treatment by several decades. Since therapeutic compliance is poor in most populations, and treatment failure has implications for the patient's sex partners, the community at large, and the patient's own health, single-dose treatment is especially important in STD management. Direct observation of treatment by the clinician or other office personnel also is important, because studies show high rates of failure to fill prescriptions and properly take the medication. Directly observed single-dose therapy is the treatment of choice for chlamydial infection, gonorrhea, chancroid, and syphilis. Even when multiple-dose regimens must be used, it is good practice to give the patient his or her antibiotic in the clinic and observe the first dose. Studies show that approximately 25% of persons treated with 7-day courses of doxycycline for chlamydial infection or acute PID fail even to fill their prescriptions, or for other reasons take little or no drug.

MANAGEMENT OF SEX PARTNERS

Management of patients' sex partners is integral to STD clinical care. With few exceptions, the partners of persons with treatable bacterial STDs should be treated presumptively, without awaiting the results of specific diagnostic tests. (Diagnostic tests should be performed, however, because the partner's understanding of the importance of compliance, follow-up, and successful treatment of any additional sex partners is contingent on documented infection.) Failure to treat the partner often is tantamount to not treating the index case, who may be reinfected, and fosters spread to additional persons.

When practical, the clinician should be available personally to examine his or her patients' sex partners. For example, reproductive health clinics must be available to evaluate and treat the male partners of their patients, and health maintenance organizations should offer services to the nonmember partners of their patients; such management is likely to be less costly than the complications that otherwise will occur in many reinfected index patients. If evaluation of the partner by the patient's own provider is not feasible, the clinician should make a specific referral to an alternate source of care; vague advice to "make sure your partner gets treated" is often unheeded.

Anecdotal reports suggest that many clinicians sometimes arrange for treatment of their patients' sex partners without examination, by writing prescriptions in the partners' names or giving patients twice the normal amount of antibiotic with instructions to share the drug with their partners. Public health officials have long condemned this practice. However, only a small number of the partners of persons with chlamydial infection, gonorrhea, or syphilis actually receive treatment when personal examination of the partners is required, even when well-funded public programs use trained staff to notify partners. Ongoing research is underway to address these issues. Until the results are available, the preferred management remains personal examination and treatment of STD patients' sex partners. Blind treatment of the partners may lead to incomplete treatment, missed opportunities to bring other partners to treatment, and may carry medicolegal risks. However, when it is clear that the partner will not otherwise be treated, such blind therapy often is appropriate.

In some geographic areas, the local or state health department will assist in partner notification for some STDs, such as syphilis, gonorrhea, HIV infection, and sometimes chlamydial infection. For most STDs, however, the clinician will need to advise his or her patients to inform their partners. Most patients need assistance in deciding which contacts need to be notified, depending on the specific infection, the date of onset, the usual incubation period, and related considerations. The process can be integrated with risk-reduction counseling.

COUNSELING

Clinicians who treat persons with STD should help their patients reduce the risk of infection in the future. Sexual safety should be addressed with all young people, using the same forthright but sensitive approach that works for taking the medical and sexual histories. Sexual abstinence and maintenance of a permanent, mutually monogamous relationship should be emphasized as the surest measures to prevent STD, as should the use of condoms for nonmonogamous sexual encounters. The extremely high rates of STD in sexually active teenagers may be more related to "serial monogamy" than to simultaneous partnerships; therefore, most unmarried persons <20 years old should use condoms for all sexual exposures, even in apparently committed relationships.

Counseling also should address selectivity in choosing sexual partners, the recognition and response to symptoms of STD, and the links between STD and substance abuse and between HIV infection and other STDs. It also is worthwhile to advise patients to avoid situations and settings that are especially conducive to high-risk sexual behavior, such as alcohol, substance abuse, and places where anonymous sexual encounters are expected. Regardless of the clinician's personal views on community standards or other aspects of sexuality, he or she should understand that most persons at risk will more readily accept education and counseling based on pragmatic rationales than on moral or religious grounds.

SCREENING AND THE ROUTINE STD CLINICAL EVALUATION

Screening means laboratory testing for STDs in persons at risk, in the absence of symptoms, signs, known STD exposure, or other clinical evidence of infection. Acquiring an STD is a "sentinel event" that reflects unprotected sexual activity. In addition to management of the patient's primary complaint, the clinical encounter should usually include testing for other common STDs. When practical, persons at risk also should be screened whenever they present for health care for any reason. The specific STDs for which such testing is indicated depends on the local prevalence of specific infections, test performance, the potential impact of case detection on patient's health, the frequency and personal and financial costs of the sequelae that might be prevented by early detection of infection, the direct cost of the test, and indirect costs, such as the convenience and time required for the test procedure. Screening has a central role in the control of chlamydial infection, gonorrhea, syphilis, and HIV infection and may prove important for the prevention of genital herpes and HPV infection. Screening recommendations for specific STDs are discussed in the chapters that follow.

Sometimes asymptomatic patients present with a request for comprehensive STD assessment. The patient's age and other factors will determine the specific laboratory tests. Because chlamydial infection is common in all settings and populations, a test for *C. trachomatis* generally should be done in both men and women, especially in persons ≤30 years old. Most such patients will request or should be offered HIV counseling and testing. With the ready availability of type-specific HSV serological tests, most patients requesting comprehensive STD screening should be offered an antibody test for HSV-2 infection. The need for gonorrhea testing depends on the local prevalence of infection and the patient's risk history; however, gonorrhea testing generally is inexpensive and usually should be offered. Women should be evaluated for the common vulvovaginal infections, which may be asymptomatic. Both men and women should have a careful inspection for warts, ulcers, and other lesions. The need for a serological test for syphilis in many heterosexual patients has declined, as the incidence of syphilis has fallen to very low levels in most of the United States; however, the test is inexpensive and many patients expect routine syphilis screening. As noted above, the need and value of a specific test for HPV remains controversial. Asymptomatic MSM who request STD evaluation generally should be tested for rectal gonorrhea and chlamydial infection, pharyngeal gonococcal infection, HIV, HSV-2 infection, and depending on past infection or immunization history, hepatitis B and hepatitis A antibody.

Finally, screening has an important role in STD prevention in outreach settings. Most patients with STD or at risk do not regularly attend physicians' offices or other traditional clinical facilities. Selected STD screening is proving to be an important prevention strategy for young persons attending school-based clinics, community centers, facilities for the evaluation and treatment of substance abuse, other social services settings, and even on the streets, in parks, or other settings where young people at risk may congregate. The development of urine-based testing and innovative methods to collect serological specimens (e.g., finger-stick testing, oral fluids) are expanding the spectrum of settings where STD screening can be implemented.

REPORTING

Data on STD morbidity and local and regional epidemiology are essential for the rational design of prevention programs and to leverage resources for public health intervention, and these resources can be directed to populations and communities at risk only if their occurrence, location, and demographic characteristics are known. Chlamydial infection, gonorrhea, syphilis, hepatitis B, and AIDS are universally reportable, and HIV infection in the absence of overt AIDS increasingly so. In addition to collating statistics and undertaking epidemiologic analysis, health departments often use STD case reports to initiate confidential partner notification. Clinicians should be familiar with local regulations and report all cases of designated STDs.

ADDITIONAL READING

Centers for Disease Control and Prevention: 1998 guidelines for treatment of sexually transmitted diseases. *MMWR* 47(RR-1):1–116, 1998. *CDC's evidence-based recommendations for treatment of STDs Revised guidelines are anticipated in 2001.*

Centers for Disease Control and Prevention: HIV prevention through early detection and treatment of other sexually transmitted diseases—United States. *MMWR* 47(No. RR 12):1–24, 1998. *CDC policy statement and recommendations on the potential contribution of STD prevention to control of HIV/AIDS.*

Eng TR, Butler WR (eds): *The Hidden Epidemic: Confronting Sexually Transmitted Diseases.* Washington, DC, National Academy Press, 1997. *A comprehensive report (432 pp) by the Institute of Medicine, National Academy of Sciences, on the epidemiology of STDs and the status of STD prevention in the United States.*

Fleming DT, Wasserheit JN: From epidemiological synergy to public health policy and practice: the contribution of other sexually transmitted diseases to transmission of HIV infection. *Sex Transm Infect* 75:3–17, 1999. *A comprehensive review of the influence of traditional STDs on HIV transmission and implications for HIV prevention.*

Garnett GP, Anderson RM: Sexually transmitted diseases and sexual behavior: insights from mathematical models. *J Infect Dis* 174:S150–S161, 1996. *A review of the mathematics of core groups in STD epidemiology.*

Holmes KK et al (ed): *Sexually Transmitted Diseases*, 3d ed. New York, McGraw-Hill, 1999. *The definitive textbook on STDs (1454 pp).*

BACTERIAL SEXUALLY TRANSMITTED DISEASES

Chapter 2
CHLAMYDIAL INFECTIONS

Chlamydia trachomatis is a small bacterium that invades eukaryotic cells and requires cell culture for isolation. Chlamydial infection is the most prevalent bacterial STD in industrialized countries and perhaps worldwide; along with genital herpes and human papillomavirus (HPV) infection, it is one of the three most common STDs in the United States. Some serotypes cause blinding trachoma, a continuing public health problem in some developing countries. Three serological variants (serovars) cause lymphogranuloma venereum (LGV), one of the five classic venereal diseases (with gonorrhea, syphilis, chancroid, and granuloma inguinale). The LGV and trachoma serovars are uncommon in industrialized countries. *Chlamydia pneumoniae* is a respiratory pathogen that has been linked with coronary artery disease and atherosclerosis; it is not sexually transmitted.

In adults, the dominant manifestations of infection with the non–LGV serovars of *C. trachomatis* are urethritis, cervicitis, proctitis, and conjunctivitis, all of which commonly are mild and often asymptomatic. This clinical spectrum is similar to that of gonorrhea, but with less florid inflammatory symptoms and signs, a longer incubation period, and more frequent subclinical infection. Paradoxically, the outwardly mild nature of chlamydial infection may enhance the frequency of complications, because treatment is often delayed and significant scarring (e.g., fallopian tube obstruction) can result from subclinical infection. The organism can be found in the upper genital tracts of most women with cervical infection, despite absence of clinical evidence of endometritis or salpingitis, and most women with tubal infertilty due to *C. trachomatis* have no past history of pelvic inflammatory disease (PID) or unexplained abdominal pain. In addition, pathophysiologic studies and epidemiologic research indicate that repeat infection is associated with a disproportionate risk of complications, probably due to a vigorous anamnestic cellular immune response. Difficulties in clinical recognition and diagnosis have seriously hampered prevention and control.

EPIDEMIOLOGY

Incidence and Prevalence Estimated annual incidence 3 million infections in the United States; in Seattle, reported infections approximate 300 per 100,000 annually overall, and 2000 per 100,000 in female teenagers 15–19 years old (i.e., 2% per year, or 4% per year in sexually active teen girls); among women aged ≤25 years, prevalence averages 5% in primary care practices and reproductive health clinics, 10–30% in STD clinics, and 5–10% in secondary school–based clinics, community centers, and social service sites; prevalence typically 5–10% in sexually active males 15–30 years; infection is now reportable in almost all states; wherever widespread screening of women has been instituted, prevalence and incidence have declined; LGV rare in the United States (average reported cases 260/year in the 1990s) and Western Europe, but remains common in some developing countries

Transmission Exclusively by sexual contact or perinatally, except for transmission of trachoma strains among children; pharyngeal infection and transmission by oral sex rare, in contrast to gonorrhea

Age Strong association with young age, probably due to both biological factors (e.g., physiologic cervical ectopy) and sexual behavior; peak incidence and prevalence age 15–19 in females, 20–24 in males

Sex More reported cases in women than men, because women are screened more frequently and many men with symptomatic infection are treated without diagnostic confirmation; true M:F incidence ratio about 1:1

Sexual Orientation Isolated less frequently in MSM than heterosexual men and women, but seroprevalence studies nonetheless suggest frequent infection in MSM; LGV occasionally causes severe proctocolitis in MSM; apparently rare in exclusively lesbian women.

Other Risk Factors Strong association with low socioeconomic and education levels and African American or Hispanic race/ethnicity; hormonal contraception associated with higher prevalence in women, but uncertain whether this reflects susceptibility or sensitivity of laboratory diagnosis.

HISTORY

Incubation Period One week to several months (usually 1–3 weeks) in symptomatic persons, but many infections remain subclinical

Symptoms In men, urethral discharge, often scant, and dysuria, usually mild, sometimes described as urethral itching or tingling; in women, vaginal discharge, dysuria, intermenstrual or postcoital vaginal bleeding, low abdominal pain; or other symptoms of urethritis, cervicitis, salpingitis, epididymitis, or conjunctivitis (see Chaps. 3, 14–19).

Epidemiologic and Exposure History Presence of STD risk factors and markers enhances risk, but infection is common in their absence; because many infections persist for months and perhaps years, recent sexual exposures often are poor predictors of infection

PHYSICAL EXAMINATION

Signs of urethritis, cervicitis, salpingitis, proctitis, epididymitis, and other manifestations (see Chaps. 14–19); mucoid or mucopurulent discharge is more common than overtly purulent exudate; often normal

LABORATORY DIAGNOSIS

Identification of the Organism DNA amplification assays using ligase chain reaction (LCR), polymerase chain reaction (PCR), or transcription-mediated amplification (TMA) detect 90–95% of infections in genital secretions or urine, and are the tests of choice; culture detects 70–80% of infections (with substantial variability among laboratories), can be performed on rectal samples but not urine; nonamplified DNA probe tests and assays to identify *C. trachomatis* antigens detect only 50–70% of infections, approved only for urethral or cervical specimens, but less expensive than other tests

Serology Antibody tests (microimmunofluorescence or complement fixation) useful in diagnosis of LGV (complement fixation titer usually ≥1:128); rarely useful in other clinical settings, but sometimes used in evaluation of female infertility

TREATMENT

Uncomplicated Infection Azithromycin 1.0 g PO, single dose, directly observed; or doxycycline 100 mg PO *bid* for 7 days, if compliance assured; each has ≥95% efficacy

Alternative Regimens Ofloxacin 300 mg PO *bid* for 7 days; erythromycin base 500 mg PO *qid* for 7 days (<90% efficacy)

Pregnant Women Amoxicillin 500 mg PO *qid* for 7–10 days; azithromycin 1.0 g PO, as above; erythromycin base, as above

LGV Doxycycline 100 mg PO *bid* for 21 days; erythromycin base 500 mg PO *qid* for 21 days

Follow-up of Uncomplicated Infection Test of cure usually not indicated following azithromycin or doxycycline, unless therapeutic compliance in question; test of cure recommended 2–3 weeks following erythromycin treatment and in all pregnant women, regardless of regimen used.

MANAGEMENT OF SEX PARTNERS

Notify, test, and treat all sex partners, regardless of symptoms or signs of infection; depending on patient's sex history, it may be necessary to notify past partners; local or state health department may assist in partner management

PREVENTION

Counseling Emphasize importance of preventing future infections, due to enhanced risk of complications, especially in women; encourage monogamy, condoms, selectivity in sex partner selection

Screening Because most infections are silent, screening sexually active young persons is central to prevention; urine testing with a DNA amplification test permits screening when genital examination impractical; test all sexually active women ≤20 years old, and those 21–30 years old if ≥1 sex partner, new partner, or symptomatic partner; also screen sexually active teen boys and young men (≤30 years old) with urine tests; all pregnant women should be tested routinely to prevent neonatal infection

Rescreening Retest women with chlamydial infection 3–4 months after treatment, because 10–20% have recurrent or persistent infection due to sexual reexposure or poor therapeutic compliance

Reporting Promptly report cases as required by local regulations

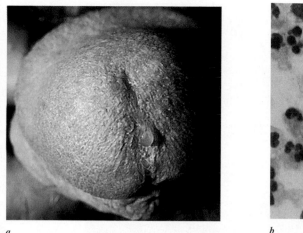
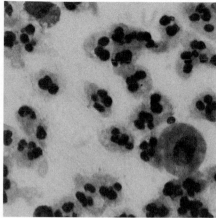

a   *b*

2–1. Nongonococcal urethritis due to *Chlamydia trachomatis*. *a.* Mucopurulent urethral discharge. *b.* Gram-stained urethral smear showing PMNs without ICGND. Compare with Figs. 3–1, 3–3*b*, 3–6, 3–8, and 17–3*b*.

Patient Profile   Age 19, single heterosexual college sophomore

History   Began new sexual relationship 6 weeks earlier; prior partnership ended 2 months ago; 3 weeks' intermittent urethral discharge without dysuria; referred by his new partner after she had positive screening test for *C. trachomatis*

Examination   Cloudy mucoid discharge expressed by urethral compression

Differential Diagnosis   Chlamydial urethritis, nonchlamydial nongonococcal urethritis (NGU); gonococcal, trichomonal, and herpetic urethritis possible but less likely

Laboratory   Urethral Gram stain showed 10–15 PMNs per 1000× field, without ICGND; cultures for *C. trachomatis* (positive) and *N. gonorrhoeae* (negative); VDRL and HIV antibody test (both negative)

Diagnosis   Chlamydial NGU

Treatment   Azithromycin 1.0 g PO, single dose, directly observed

Sex Partner Management   Advised to refer former girlfriend, but patient declined; local health department contacted for assistance in locating and arranging for diagnosis and treatment

Comment   Mild symptoms resulted in delayed care until his partner's chlamydial infection was diagnosed, a common sequence of events

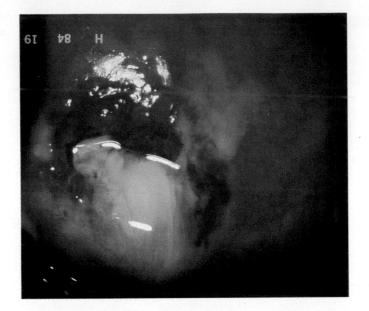

2–2. Mucopurulent cervicitis due to *Chlamydia trachomatis* (see also Figs 3–2, 17–1a, 17–3, etc). (Courtesy of Claire E. Stevens.)

Patient Profile   Age 17 years old, high school junior

History   Asymptomatic; presented to a public health family planning clinic for refill of her oral contraceptive prescription; sexually active for 6 weeks with a single male partner, a local college student; a prior relationship, with a high school classmate, ended 2 months previously

Examination   Mucopurulent exudate emanating from cervical os; small area of edematous cervical ectopy; swab-induced endocervical bleeding

Differential Diagnosis   Mucopurulent cervicitis due to *C. trachomatis* or *N. gonorrhoeae;* rule out trichomoniasis and other cervicovaginal infections

Laboratory   Cervical Gram stain showed 15–20 PMNs per 1000× field, without ICGND; vaginal fluid pH 4.0 with negative KOH amine odor test; no yeast, clue cells, or trichomonads seen on KOH and saline wet mounts; cervical LCR test for *C. trachomatis* (positive); cervical culture for *N. gonorrhoeae* (negative); serologic tests for syphilis and HIV (negative)

Diagnosis   Asymptomatic mucopurulent cervicitis due to *C. trachomatis*

Treatment   Azithromycin 1.0 g PO, single dose, directly observed

Follow-up   Advised to return 3 months later to provide a urine specimen for a rescreening LCR test

Sex Partner Management   Advised to refer both male partners for diagnosis and treatment

Comment   Overt cervicitis was present despite lack of symptoms; test of cure not routinely recommended, but rescreening indicated 3–4 months after treatment to detect both persistent and recurrent infection

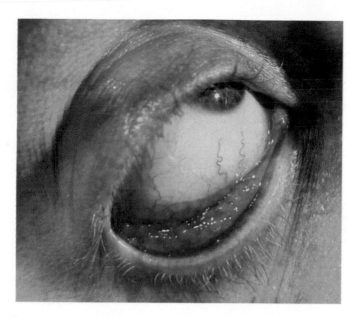

2–3. Chlamydial conjunctivitis (compare with gonococcal conjunctivitis, Fig. 3–3).

Patient Profile   Age 22, female flight attendant

History   Mild itching of eyes for 2–3 weeks; boyfriend was treated a month earlier for "urinary tract infection"; no other sex partners in the past year

Examination   Slight conjunctival erythema with hypertrophied, "cobblestone" appearance; genital examination normal, without evidence of cervicitis

Differential Diagnosis   Conjunctivitis due to *C. trachomatis, N. gonorrhoeae, Haemophilus* species, other pyogenic bacteria, viruses, or allergy; rule out cervical *C. trachomatis* infection

Laboratory   Gram-stained conjunctival smear showed few mononuclear cells, rare PMNs, and no bacteria; *C. trachomatis* isolated by culture from conjunctival scraping and cervix

Diagnosis   Chlamydial conjunctivitis and asymptomatic cervical chlamydial infection

Treatment   Doxycycline 100 mg PO *bid* for 7 days

Follow-up   Advised to return after 3 months for rescreening with urine chlamydia ligase chain reaction (LCR) test

Sex Partner Management   Advised to refer her partner for retreatment because his prior antibiotic therapy was unknown and they continued unprotected intercourse after treatment; when patient said there was "no way" he would come in, she was provided with a 1.0-g dose of azithromycin to be taken by the partner

Comment   Compare with gonococcal conjunctivitis, Fig. 3–3; probably acquired either through autoinoculation or orogenital exposure; normal cervix and absence of genital symptoms are typical of chlamydial infection; patient-delivered partner therapy was judged the only likely way partner would be treated

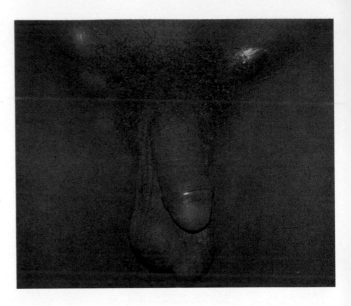

2–4. Lymphogranuloma venereum. Note separation of right lymph nodes by the inguinal ligament ("groove sign"). The left inguinal node had ruptured spontaneously. (Courtesy of Professor Olu Osoba.)

Patient Profile Age 27, unmarried man who immigrated from Ethiopia 3 weeks earlier; in Ethiopia, regularly visited commercial sex workers

History Painful swellings in groin for 3 weeks; the left swelling opened and began to drain 1 week earlier

Examination Moderately tender, firm inguinal lymphadenopathy bilaterally with firm, moderately tender nodes, 1.5–3 cm in diameter; left inguinal node had central softening and an overlying eschar; right nodes divided by inguinal ligament; no urethral discharge, genital lesions, or skin rash

Differential Diagnosis Lymphogranuloma venereum, chancroid, pyogenic infection, cat-scratch disease; liquefaction and drainage make syphilis and herpes unlikely; rule out tuberculous lymphadenitis, lymphoma, and HIV-related opportunistic diseases

Laboratory Urethral Gram stain negative for PMNs and ICGND; urethral culture for *N. gonorrhoeae* and urine LCR for *C. trachomatis* (both negative); stat RPR, routine VDRL, and HIV serology (all negative); lymph node aspirate showed overt pus, without organisms on Gram stain; few *Staphylococcus epidermidis* isolated, negative culture for *C. trachomatis;* chlamydia/LGV complement fixation test positive, titer 1:1024

Diagnosis Lymphogranuloma venereum

Treatment Doxycycline 100 mg orally *bid* for 3 weeks

Follow-up Repeated needle aspiration of left inguinal node (3 times over 8 days); repeat VDRL and HIV serology after 3 months

Sex Partner Management Patient denied identifiable sex partners

Comment Absence of detectable cutaneous primary lesion or urethritis is typical of LGV; division of involved lymph nodes by the inguinal ligament ("groove sign") is classic but seen in a minority of cases; repeated needle aspiration of fluctuant nodes may help prevent spontaneous rupture and secondary infection

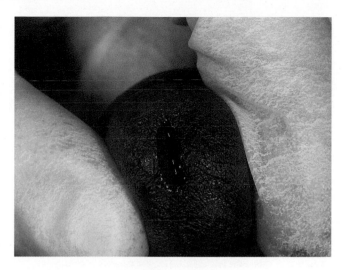

2–5. Nongonococcal urethritis due to *C. trachomatis*, with atypical blood-tinged urethral discharge

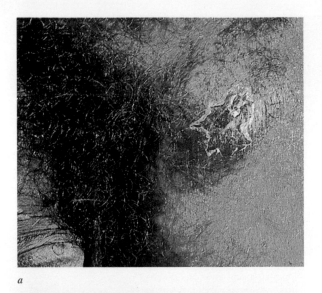

a

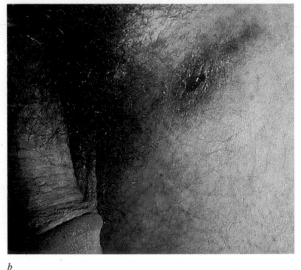

b

2–6. Probable lymphogranuloma venereum. *a.* Fluctuant femoral lymphadenopathy at presentation. *b.* Improvement after 10 days treatment with doxycycline 100 mg orally *bid.* Femoral involvement is atypical in LGV and *C. trachomatis* was not isolated from lymph node aspirate or urethra. However, the LGV complement fixation titer was reactive at a titer of 1:512. Patient also had 2 papular warts on penile shaft.

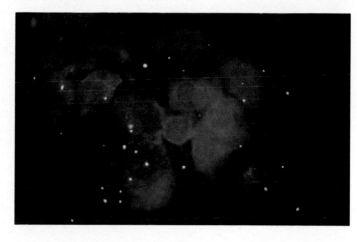

2–7. Direct immunofluorescence stain of *Chlamydia trachomatis* in an endocervical smear. *C. trachomatis* elementary bodies show bright apple-green fluorescence and host cells are counterstained red. (Courtesy of Walter E. Stamm, M.D.)

ADDITIONAL READING

Lee H et al: Diagnosis of *Chlamydia trachomatis* genitourinary infection in women by ligase chain reaction assay of urine. *Lancet* 345:213–216, 1995. *Documentation of the performance of the LCR test and sensitivity near that of cervical sampling.*

Perine PL, Stamm WE: Lymphogranuloma venereum, in *Sexually Transmitted Diseases*, 3rd ed, KK Holmes et al (eds). New York, McGraw-Hill, 1999, Chap. 30. *An excellent general review of the epidemiology and clinical aspects of LGV.*

Scholes D et al: Prevention of pelvic inflammatory disease by screening for cervical chlamydial infection. *N Engl J Med* 334:1362–1366, 1996. *A prospective study documenting reduced incidence of PID in women screened for chlamydial infection.*

Stamm WE: *Chlamydia trachomatis* infections of the adult, in *Sexually Transmitted Diseases*, 3rd ed, KK Holmes et al (eds). New York, McGraw-Hill, 1999, Chap 29. *A comprehensive, extensively referenced state-of-the-art review.*

Chapter 3
GONORRHEA

Gonorrhea is among the most common and most widely recognized sexually transmitted diseases (STDs) throughout the world. *Neisseria gonorrhoeae*, a Gram-negative diplococcus that in clinical material typically appears within polymorphonuclear leukocytes (PMNs), primarily affects the mucosal surfaces of the urethra or endocervix and secondarily those of the rectum, pharynx, and conjunctivae. Ascending infection in women results in gonococcal pelvic inflammatory disease (PID), the most common complication and an important cause of female infertility. Bacteremic dissemination causes a characteristic arthritis–dermatitis syndrome and rarely bacterial endocarditis or meningitis. Other complications are acute epididymitis and, in infants born to infected mothers, blindness resulting from conjunctivitis (ophthalmia neonatorum) that leads to corneal scarring. Transmission occurs almost exclusively through sexual or perinatal exposure.

EPIDEMIOLOGY

Incidence Incidence declining in the United States since the late 1970s; 355,000 cases reported (estimated 700,000 total) in 1998, or 133 cases per 100,000 population, the lowest since statistics first tabulated in the 1930s; reported incidence varies widely, with most cases occurring in low socioeconomic populations because of high frequencies of illicit drug use and commercial sex, and in MSM; highest rates persist in southeastern states

Prevalence Varies widely, based on local and regional incidence; 5–20% of patients in many urban STD clinics and some corrections facilities; now generally <1% of sexually active women in private physicians' offices and most reproductive health clinics; rising in MSM in some cities

Transmission Most cases acquired through vaginal or anal intercourse, 20–50% transmission risk per unprotected exposure; orogenital contact less efficient, especially from pharynx to genitals, but oral sex explains an increasing proportion of urethral gonorrhea in MSM

Age All ages susceptible; almost 80% of cases occur in females aged 15–29 and males aged 15–34 years; median age several years older than for chlamydial infection

Sex Male:female ratio approximately 1:1 to 1:2; varies with success of case-finding in asymptomatic women, frequency of commercial sex in the community, and proportion of cases occurring in MSM

Sexual Orientation Dramatic decline in cases in MSM from early 1980s until mid-1990s, then rising incidence in MSM in late 1990s, possibly due to relaxed attitudes toward AIDS in response to HIV treatment advances; annual gonorrhea rate in MSM remains several times higher than in heterosexuals; apparently rare in exclusively homosexual women

Other Risk Markers Unmarried marital status; lower educational and socioeconomic levels; illicit drug use; prostitution, previous gonorrhea; low rates of condom use; rates several times higher in African Americans and Hispanics than in whites or most Asian populations

HISTORY

Incubation Period Typically 2–5 days for urethritis in men, 5–10 days in women; 1–5% of urethral infections in men and 20–40% of cervical infections remain subclinical for prolonged periods; incubation variable for symptoms of PID, proctitis, and disseminated infections; most rectal and almost all pharyngeal infections remain asymptomatic

Symptoms In men, urethral discharge, often large in amount, with or without dysuria; in women, any combination of vaginal discharge, dysuria, intermenstrual bleeding, low abdominal pain, or other symptoms of urethritis, cervicitis, salpingitis, epididymitis, or conjunctivitis (see Chaps. 2, 14–19); symptoms usually more prominent than for chlamydial infection; symptomatic proctitis causes anal discharge, pruritus, occasionally tenesmus and rectal bleeding; occasional sore throat; major symptoms of complications are low abdominal pain, testicular pain and swelling, polyarthralgia, arthritis, skin lesions, conjunctival pain and discharge, constitutional symptoms

Epidemiologic and Exposure History Infection uncommon in absence of behavioral risk factors and demographic markers (unlike chlamydial infection); most patients acknowledge new sex partner or partner known to have other partners

PHYSICAL EXAMINATION

Urethritis in Men Urethral discharge, usually overt but sometimes demonstrated only by "milking" urethra; discharge usually opaque, white or yellow in color, but sometimes mucoid or mucopurulent; occasional meatal erythema; rarely penile edema or overt lymphangitis; may be normal

Urogential Infection in Women Purulent or mucopurulent endocervical exudate or other signs of mucopurulent cervicitis (see Chap. 17); sometimes purulent exudate expressible from urethra, periurethral (Skene's) glands, or Bartholin gland duct; occasional uterine or adnexal tenderness or mass (see Chap. 19); may be normal

Rectal Infection Usually normal; occasional perianal erythema; anoscopy may show mucosal erythema, punctate bleeding, purulent exudate

Pharyngeal Infection Usually normal; rare erythema, purulent exudate, cervical lymphadenopathy

LABORATORY DIAGNOSIS

Gram-Stained Smear Polymorphonuclear leukocytes (PMNs) with intracellular gram-negative diplococci (ICGND); both sensitive and specific in symptomatic urethritis; for cervical, rectal, or asymptomatic urethral infection, detects <50% of cases, although clearly positive result is reliable indicator of gonorrhea; not useful in pharyngeal infection

Culture Culture on selective growth medium detects ≥95% of male urethral gonorrhea and 80–90% of cervical, rectal, and pharyngeal infections; culture is test of choice in most settings and the only method that permits antimicrobial susceptibility testing

Other Tests Nonculture tests are increasingly sensitive and specific; DNA amplification tests,

including ligase chain reaction (LCR), polymerase chain reaction (PCR), and transcription-mediated amplification (TMA) sensitivities comparable to culture and retain sensitivity on urine; nonamplified DNA probe tests and antigen detection assays are less sensitive, and false-positive results may be common in low-prevalence settings; no nonculture test is approved for rectal or pharyngeal specimens

TREATMENT

Principles Penicillin-resistant *N. gonorrhoeae* strains are prevalent worldwide, and strains with other kinds of antibiotic resistance continue to evolve and spread; gonococci with high-level resistance to fluoroquinolones now are common in parts of Asia, but to date uncommon in the United States; significant cephalosporin resistance has not evolved; treat with single-dose regimen plus therapy for *Chlamydia trachomatis* infection, present in 15–30% of heterosexual men and women, but ≤ 5% of MSM; combination treatment may also retard selection of antibiotic-resistant gonococci; all initial single-dose regimens are equally effective

Uncomplicated Gonorrhea in Adults

INITIAL SINGLE-DOSE, DIRECTLY OBSERVED TREATMENT

- Cefixime 400 mg PO
- Ceftriaxone 125 mg IM
- Ciprofloxacin 500 mg PO
- Ofloxacin 400 mg PO

FOLLOW-UP TREATMENT

- Azithromycin 1.0 g PO, single dose
- Doxycycline 100 mg PO *bid* for 7 days

Pregnant Women Avoid ciprofloxacin, ofloxacin, and doxycycline; if cephalosporins contraindicated (e.g., allergy), use spectinomycin 2.0 g IM, single dose; for follow-up antichlamydial therapy, use amoxicillin, azithromycin, or erythromycin (see Chap. 2)

Disseminated Gonococcal Infection Ceftriaxone 1.0 g IM or IV every 24 h, or ciprofloxacin 500 mg IV every 12 h, for 1–2 days or until improved; then cefixime 400 mg PO *bid*, ciprofloxacin 500 mg PO *bid*, or ofloxacin 400 mg PO *bid*, to complete 7 days total therapy

Follow-up Test-of-cure not indicated following directly observed therapy of uncomplicated gonorrhea with recommended regimens;

women should be rescreened for *N. gonorrhoeae* and *C. trachomatis* 2–4 months after treatment

MANAGEMENT OF SEX PARTNERS

Notify, test, and treat all sex partners in the 2–4 weeks prior to acquisition; local or state health department may assist in locating partners

PREVENTION

Counseling Emphasize importance of preventing future infections and assuring treatment of partners; encourage monogamy, condoms, selectivity in sex partner selection; emphasize the strong epidemiologic and behavioral link between bacterial STDs and risk of HIV infection; many patients require advice or assistance with referral for substance abuse treatment

Screening Routinely test women in population groups and settings with high rates of gonorrhea; screening heterosexual men of uncertain value, because asymptomatic urethral infection is rare; screen MSM at risk for rectal and pharyngeal infection

Reporting Report cases according to local regulations; some health departments request immediate reporting by telephone

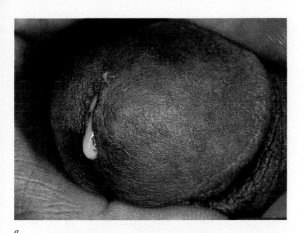

a

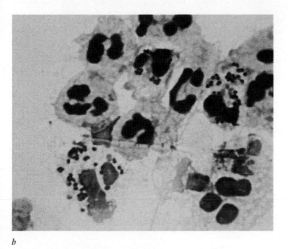

b

3–1. Gonococcal urethritis. *a.* Purulent urethral discharge. *b.* Gram-stained smear showing intracellular gram-negative diplococci. Compare with Fig. 2–1.

Patient Profile   Age 22, carwash attendant

History   Urethral discharge for 1 day, mild dysuria; intercourse with a new female partner 4 days earlier and with regular girlfriend 2 days ago

Examination   Copious purulent urethral discharge; otherwise normal

Differential Diagnosis   Gonorrhea, nongonococcal urethritis

Laboratory   PMNs with ICGND on urethral smear; cultures for *N. gonorrhoeae* and *C. trachomatis* (both positive); VDRL and HIV serology (both negative)

Diagnosis   Gonococcal urethritis (with chlamydial infection)

Treatment   Cefixime 400 mg PO plus azithromycin 1.0 g PO (both single dose, directly observed)

Follow-up   Scheduled for HIV post-test counseling after 7 days, but failed to return

Sex Partner Management   Following interview by health department counselor, both recent partners were located, examined, and treated; new partner had gonorrhea, regular partner culture-negative

Comment   From 10 to 15% of heterosexual men with gonorrhea also have urethral *C. trachomatis* infection

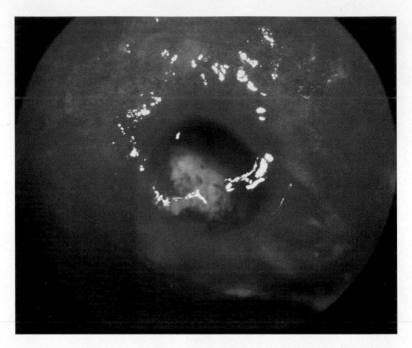

3–2. Gonococcal cervicitis, with scant purulent exudate in os. (Courtesy of King K. Holmes, M.D., Ph.D.)

Patient Profile   Age 18, new partner of preceding patient

History   Asymptomatic; no other partners in past 4 months; had "hives" after receiving penicillin during childhood

Examination   Mucopurulent cervical exudate; otherwise normal

Differential Diagnosis   Mucopurulent cervicitis; epidemiologic information suggests gonorrhea; 20–30% probability of concomitant chlamydial infection

Laboratory   Gram stain of cervical exudate showed PMNs without ICGND; cervical cultures for *N. gonorrhoeae* and *C. trachomatis* (both positive); VDRL and HIV serology negative

Diagnosis   Gonococcal cervicitis (with chlamydial infection)

Treatment   Ciprofloxacin 500 mg PO, single dose, directly observed; plus doxycycline 100 mg orally *bid* for 7 days

Follow-up   Scheduled for HIV post-test counseling (7 days) and returned as scheduled; advised to return again in 3 months to provide urine for LCR testing for *N. gonorrhoeae* and *C. trachomatis*

Sex Partner Management   Already treated

Comment   Ciprofloxacin selected over cefixime or ceftriaxone because of history suggesting type I allergic reaction to penicillin; patient was judged reliable for compliance with doxycycline for 7 days; counseled to use condoms consistently

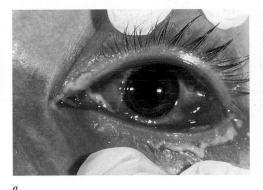 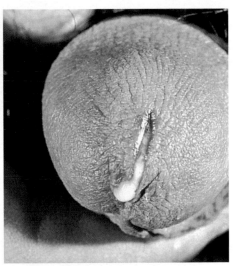

a

3–3. *a.* Gonococcal conjunctivitis; compare with chlamydial conjunctivitis (Fig. 2–3).
b. Gonococcal urethritis.

Patient Profile　Age 33, gay, computer programmer

History　Urethral discharge 3 days; left eye pain and photophobia 2 days; one regular sex partner, plus frequent anonymous partnerships with other men at bath houses; HIV negative when tested 3 months previously

Examination　Conjunctival erythema and purulent exudate, subconjunctival hemorrhage; purulent urethral discharge

Differential Diagnosis　Urethritis, probably gonorrhea, rule out chlamydial infection; purulent conjunctivitis, rule out *N. gonorrhoeae,* other pyogenic bacteria, herpes simplex virus (HSV), *C. trachomatis*

Laboratory　PMNs with ICGND in both conjunctival and urethral exudate; cultures from both sites positive for *N. gonorrhoeae*; urethral and conjunctival cultures negative for *C. trachomatis* and HSV; rectal and pharyngeal cultures negative for *N. gonorrhoeae*; rectal culture negative for *C. trachomatis*; VDRL negative; declined HIV testing

Diagnosis　Gonococcal urethritis and conjunctivitis

Treatment　Cefixime 400 mg PO daily for 7 days, first dose directly observed

Follow-up　Scheduled to return after 2 days and 1 week to assess conjunctivitis

Sex Partner Management　Patient notified regular partner, who was treated by his private physician

Comment　Compare with chlamydial conjunctivitis (Fig. 2–3); conjunctivitis may have resulted from autoinoculation from his own urethral infection, or from direct oropharyngeal exposure from a sex partner; gonococcal conjunctivitis is treated for ≥7 days; antichlamydial therapy is optional, because fewer MSM than heterosexuals with gonorrhea are co-infected; counseling emphasized the high risk of HIV associated with patient's sexual behavior

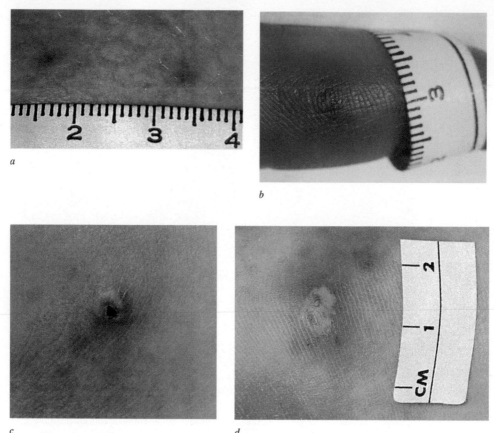

3–4. Skin lesions in gonococcal arthritis–dermatitis syndrome. *a.* Early papular lesions of forearm. *b.* Hemorrhagic lesion of finger. *c.* Pustule with central eschar. *d.* Large hemorrhagic pustule of foot. (Parts *a* and *b* are from the patient described. Parts *c* and *d* are from two other patients.) Lesions typically begin as nonspecific papules or petechiae, then progress to pustules, often with a hemorrhagic component. The rulers in parts *a, b,* and *d* are metric.

Patient Profile   Age 22, female, "exotic" dancer

History   Generalized arthralgias and "red bumps" on arms and legs for 2 days; overt pain of several joints for 1 day; intermittent vaginal discharge, without recent change; currently menstruating; refused to give information about sex partners

Examination   Afebrile; 15–20 papular, pustular, and hemorrhagic skin lesions on extremities; slight erythema and edema over left wrist, extending to dorsum of hand; pain on range of motion of left ankle, without visible abnormality; moderate effusion of right knee, with 20 mL slightly cloudy, straw-colored fluid withdrawn by needle aspiration; menstrual blood in vaginal vault, genital exam otherwise normal; normal cardiac examination

Differential Diagnosis   Disseminated gonococcal infection, Reiter's syndrome, hepatitis B prodrome, other immune complex syndromes, bacterial endocarditis, acute rheumatic fever, systemic lupus erythematosus, other acute arthritis

Laboratory   Cervical smear showed few PMNs, no ICGND; synovial fluid contained 8,500 leukocytes per mm^3, 80% PMNs, no crystals, no bacteria by Gram stain; cultures for *N. gonorrhoeae* obtained from cervix, anal canal, pharynx, synovial fluid, and blood ($\times$3); cervical culture negative for *C. trachomatis*; CBC showed 12,400 leukocytes, 80% PMNs, otherwise normal; chemistry panel normal, including liver function tests; VDRL, HIV, and hepatitis B serologies negative; *N. gonorrhoeae* isolated from cervix and pharynx; other cultures negative

Diagnosis   Disseminated gonococcal infection with arthritis–dermatitis syndrome

Treatment   Ceftriaxone 1.0 g IM, repeated 1 day later; then ofloxacin 300 mg PO *bid* for 8 days (10 days total therapy)

Follow-up   Followed daily for 3 days, then at completion of therapy; arthritis improved within 1 day and resolved by day 5; skin lesions were healed at 10 days

Sex Partner Management   In response to telephoned case report, health department counselor reinterviewed patient, without success in identifying partners

Comment   Onset of DGI during or near menses is typical; synovial fluid cultures usually are negative in arthritis–dermatitis phase, but often positive if overt septic arthritis supervenes; blood cultures may be positive or negative; careful cardiac examination and close follow-up indicated for first 2–3 days, because 1–3% of patients have gonococcal endocarditis; ofloxacin selected for completion of therapy because of efficacy against both *N. gonorrhoeae* and *C. trachomatis*; gonococcal strains most likely to cause DGI are now uncommon in the United States

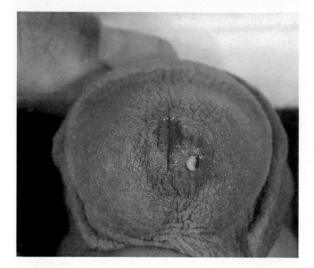

3–5. Periurethral furuncle due to
N. gonorrhoeae. Patient presented
with history of "pimple" at tip of
penis, draining intermittently for 6
weeks, without urethral discharge or
dysuria. Gram stain of expressed
exudate showed PMNs with ICGND,
culture positive for *N. gonorrhoeae*.

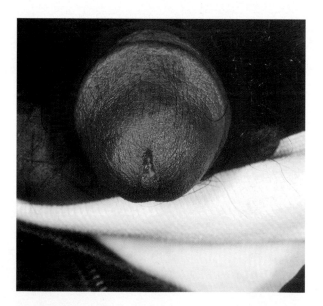

3–6. Scant mucopurulent exudate
in gonococcal urethritis; not all cases
have opaque, overtly purulent
discharge *(compare with Figs. 3–1
and 3–3b)*.

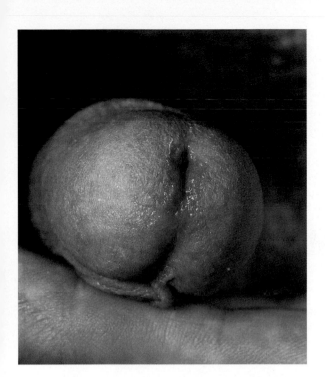

3–7. Gonococcal urethritis manifested by scant, clear urethral discharge and urethral erythema; ICGND were present on Gram-stained smear and *N. gonorrhoeae* was isolated.

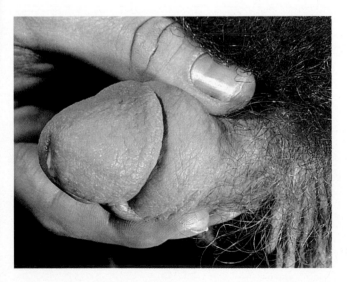

3–8. Gonococcal urethritis with distal penile edema ("bull-headed clap"); this rare manifestation has also been termed "penile venereal edema" and can also occur with genital herpes *(Fig. 7–6)* or NGU. *(Fig. 14–3).*

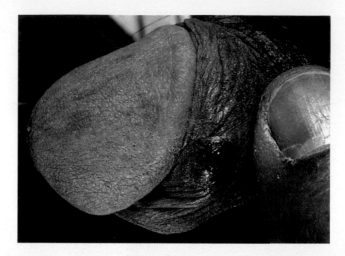

3–9. Presumptive gonococcal ulcer of the penis in a patient with gonococcal urethritis; *N. gonorrhoeae* was isolated from the ulcer as well as the urethra; darkfield microscopy, syphilis serology, and cultures for HSV and *Haemophilus ducreyi* were negative. *N. gonorrhoeae* is a rare cause of ulceration of the genitals or fingers; most cases probably represent secondary gonococcal infection of preexisting skin lesions.

ADDITIONAL READING

Handsfield HH, Whittington WL: Antibiotic-resistant *Neisseria gonorrhoeae*: the calm before another storm? [Editorial]. *Ann Intern Med* 125:507–508, 1996. *A commentary on fluoroquinolone resistance and the potential for future spread in the United States.*

Holmes KK et al: Disseminated gonococcal infection. *Ann Intern Med* 74:979–993, 1971. *An older paper, still the classic modern description of disseminated gonococcal infection.*

Hook EW III, Handsfield HH: Gonococcal infections in the adult, in *Sexually Transmitted Diseases*, 3rd ed, KK Holmes et al (eds). New York, McGraw-Hill, 1999, Chap 32. *A comprehensive, state-of-the-art review.*

Moran JS, Handsfield HH: *Neisseria gonorrhoeae,* in *Antimicrobial Therapy and Vaccines,* VL Yu et al (eds). Baltimore, Williams & Wilkins, 1999, pp 295–303. *Review of treatment options for gonorrhea, with emphasis on studies conducted since 1990.*

Chapter 4
SYPHILIS

Syphilis has been recognized since the late fifteenth century. It is characterized by a complex natural history that is largely determined by the unique character of the causative spirochete, *Treponema pallidum,* and the immunologic response to it. The pathogenesis is similar to that of tuberculosis. Both infections are caused by slowly replicating pathogens whose containment depends on cell-mediated immunity; both are distinguished by an apparently benign primary infection accompanied by silent bacteremia with dissemination of organisms to various organs. In both diseases destructive granulomatous inflammation results if infection reactivates, sometimes due to acquired immunodeficiency.

Syphilis is classically described as having distinct primary, secondary, and tertiary stages over several years or decades, interspersed by periods of inactive ("latent") infection. These distinctions, however, are sometimes blurred; for example, neurosyphilis, often considered a manifestation of tertiary infection, commonly occurs in early syphilis. Blunted responses to antibiotic therapy, aberrant results of serological tests for syphilis, and an increased risk of neurosyphilis have been reported in HIV-infected persons with syphilis, but appear to be uncommon.

The incidence of infectious (primary, secondary, and early latent) syphilis has fluctuated widely in the United States over the past 5 decades. Reported rates rose in the 1970s and early 1980s, largely due to increased cases in gay and bisexual men, but both overall incidence and rates in men who have sex with men (MSM) declined rapidly after the mid-1980s as a result of behavioral changes in response to AIDS. Early syphilis rates again rose rapidly in the late 1980s, primarily in heterosexual populations with high incidences of illicit drug use and social disruption. During the 1990s, the incidence of infectious syphilis declined to the lowest level at any time since national statistics were complied, and in 1999 the Centers for Disease Control and Prevention (CDC) announced plans to attempt to entirely eliminate transmission of syphilis in the United States. In some geographic areas, however, a remarkable increase in cases occurred from 1998 through 2000 among MSM, many of whom were also infected with HIV. This occurrence and the historically cyclical nature of the disease imply a clear risk for resurgent syphilis nationally.

EPIDEMIOLOGY

Incidence In the United States 6,993 cases of primary and secondary syphilis reported in 1998, or 2.6 per 100,000, the lowest in recorded history; 78% of counties reported no cases in 1998

Transmission Sexually transmissible only during primary, secondary, and early latent stages; congenital syphilis results from transplacental infection; rare cases of nonsexual transmission, sometimes in nosocomial settings

Age All ages susceptible, but most infections acquired in persons 21–34 years old (often older than persons with chlamydial infection or gonorrhea); late syphilis often diagnosed in older persons

Sex Sex distribution reflects sexual orientation and frequency of prostitution in populations at risk; slight male predominance among reported cases

Sexual Orientation Syphilis in MSM usually associated with anonymous partnerships, often in bath houses or other semipublic venues; rare in exclusively homosexual women

Other Risk Factors Illicit drug use; prostitution; low socioeconomic and educational attainment; other indirect markers of behavioral risks

CLINICAL MANIFESTATIONS

Epidemiologic and Exposure History Almost all persons with infectious syphilis acknowledge new sex partner or partner with other relationships; unprotected sex, especially with anonymous partners or with prostitutes

Incubation Period Usually 2–6 weeks (occasionally up to 3 months) from exposure to clinically evident primary syphilis

Symptoms and Examination

PRIMARY SYPHILIS Chancre often presents as a single painless or minimally painful round or oval ulcer, typically indurated, with a "clean" base (i.e., little or no purulent exudate); presence of classic chancre is insensitive but highly specific for diagnosis of syphilis; most chancres occur on external genitals, but intravaginal or perianal lesions also are common, and oral chancres occur occasionally; regional lymphadenopathy is common, generally bilateral, with firm, non-fluctuant, nontender or mildly tender nodes, without overlying erythema; usually no systemic symptoms; asymptomatic infection is common, probably due to unrecognized chancre (e.g., vaginal, anal, or rectal); all clinical manifestations and course may be highly variable, and atypical cases are common

SECONDARY SYPHILIS Protean manifestations; most common presentation is generalized papulosquamous, nonpruritic skin rash, typically including palms and soles; atypical rashes, including pruritic ones, may occur; other common manifestations include mucous patches (painless mucous membrane lesions), condylomata lata (genital or perianal warty excrescences), patchy ("moth-eaten") alopecia of the scalp, generalized lymphadenopathy, fever, headache, malaise; focal neurological manifestations, especially cranial nerve abnormalities, occur occasionally

TERTIARY (LATE) SYPHILIS Classic tertiary syphilis is rare; most common features are locally destructive granulomatous lesions (gummas) of the skin, liver, bones, or other organs; signs of late neurosyphilis include tabes dorsalis and dementia, often with paranoid features ("general paresis"); and cardiovascular manifestations, especially ascending aortic aneurysm and aortic valve insufficiency

LATENT SYPHILIS By definition, latent syphilis is asymptomatic infection that follows primary syphilis; only detectable serologically; subdivided into early-latent (infectious, ≤1 year) and late-latent (>1 year, usually noninfectious) stages

CONGENITAL SYPHILIS Severity ranges from asymptomatic to fatal; common early manifes-
tations are spontaneous abortion, stillbirth, encephalitis, generalized skin rash, rhinitis ("snuffles"), hepatic dysfunction, consumption coagulopathy, multiple organ failure; later manifestations, usually not apparent at birth, include osteitis of long bones, maxillofacial and dental malformations, keratitis, neurosensory hearing loss, and chronic neuropsychological deficits

LABORATORY DIAGNOSIS

Identification of *T. pallidum* Detection depends on visual or antigenic detection; organism diameter is smaller than light microscope resolution, requiring darkfield or phase microscopy, special stains (e.g., silver), or immunologic enhancement (e.g., immunofluorescence)

DARKFIELD MICROSCOPY Identification of motile spirochetes typical of *T. pallidum* (10 to 13 μm length, one spiral turn per μm, characteristic rotational motility and flexion) in saline-mounted scrapings from chancre or lesion of secondary syphilis, or in lymph node aspirate; frequent colonization with commensal spiral organisms limits utility for oral mucosal lesions

IMMUNOLOGIC AND GENETIC DETECTION Polyclonal fluorescent antibody test is specific and moderately sensitive substitute for darkfield microscopy; sensitive and specific fluorescent mononclonal antibody and polymerase chain reaction (PCR) assays have been developed, but to date not commercially available

HISTOLOGY Silver stain or immunofluorescence in fixed pathologic specimens; insensitive but specific, sometimes diagnostic

Serology Mainstay of laboratory diagnosis in most settings, especially after primary syphilis or when microscopy negative

NONTREPONEMAL TESTS Venereal Disease Research Laboratory (VDRL) test and variants, including rapid plasma reagin (RPR); detects antibody to cardiolipin, a component of normal mammalian cell membranes; sensitive, but nonspecific; positive results require confirmation with a treponemal antibody test

The primary uses of the nontreponemal tests are (1) screening and (2) assessment of disease activity. The VDRL or RPR becomes reactive during primary syphilis; about 70% of persons with primary syphilis have positive tests, depending on duration of symptoms when the test is obtained. Virtually all untreated patients have reactive tests after the primary stage. Reactivity rises to maximum titer (usually 1:16 to 1:256) in secondary syphilis. The titer falls spontaneously thereafter, typically to 1:1 to 1:8 in untreated late-latent infection, but often rises again if there is progression to tertiary syphilis. Reactivity declines following successful treatment. For primary and secondary syphilis, the titer should fall by 2 or more dilutions (e.g., 1:16 to 1:4) within 3 months of treatment, and in >90% of patients the test will be negative by 12 months. In late syphilis, by contrast, low titers (usually 1:1 to 1:2) often persist after apparently successful treatment. Biological false-positive results (i.e., reactive VDRL or RPR with negative treponemal test results) occasionally occur, often associated with pregnancy or immunologic disorders; the titer usually is 1:8 or lower.

TREPONEMAL ANTIBODY TESTS Tests to detect specific antibody to *T. pallidum*, such as the fluorescent treponemal antibody-absorbed (FTA-ABS) test, the microhemagglutination assay for *T. pallidum* (MHA-TP) (both of which are now less widely available), and *Treponema pallidum* particle agglutination (TPPA).

Most treponemal tests are not subject to accurate quantitation, and their primary use is to confirm positive VDRL or RPR results. In patients with secondary or later syphilis, the treponemal tests usually remain positive indefinitely, even after successful treatment, but they revert to negative in up to 25% of persons treated for primary syphilis. Once a treponemal antibody test is positive, repeat testing rarely is indicated; only the quantitative nontreponemal tests are used to monitor disease activity. Similarly, the treponemal tests are rarely if ever indicated in the presence of a negative result for VDRL or RPR; beyond the primary stage, active, clinically significant syphilis is rare if the VDRL or RPR test is negative.

DIAGNOSIS

Most cases of primary and secondary syphilis are readily suspected on clinical grounds, and the diagnosis is confirmed by laboratory tests. In contrast, diagnosis of late or latent syphilis depends primarily on serological testing. The diagnosis of syphilis is rarely if ever warranted in the absence of a reactive treponemal antibody test, except early in the primary stage. Although syphilis is increasingly rare in most clinical settings, the nontreponemal tests are inexpensive,

and when combined with treponemal confirmatory testing, false-positive results are very rare. Screening VDRL or RPR tests should continue to be used liberally in settings where syphilis persists and in selected populations at high risk for the disease.

CEREBROSPINAL FLUID EXAMINATION Neurosyphilis is the most common complication of syphilis, and many cases are subclinical. CSF examination is the primary diagnostic tool. Indications for CSF examination are neurological symptoms or signs in persons with syphilis of any stage or duration, as well as failure to respond to appropriate antibiotic therapy (because treatment failure often results from re-dissemination of *T. pallidum* sequestered in the central nervous system). For patients with syphilis >1 year in duration, indications for CSF examination are VDRL or RPR titer ≥1:32; HIV infection; other signs or symptoms of active syphilis; or planned treatment with an antibiotic other than penicillin.

TREATMENT

Principles Penicillin G remains the drug of choice for all stages of syphilis. The tetracyclines are less active against *T. pallidum* but usually are used when penicillin cannot be given. Erythromycin is still less satisfactory and is no longer recommended. The tetracyclines and erythromycin should be used only if compliance and follow-up are assured. Ceftriaxone sometimes is used when penicillin cannot be given. Azithromycin may be an effective alternative, permitting prolonged oral therapy and infrequent dosing, but experience is limited. Most other antibiotic classes have no antitreponemal activity. Antibiotic levels sufficient to inhibit *T. pallidum* should be maintained in blood and infected tissues for ≥10 days for early syphilis and ≥4 weeks for late syphilis.

Many patients with early syphilis and a few with late syphilis experience Jarisch-Herxheimer reactions, with fever, chills, malaise, headache, and sometimes increased prominence of the chancre, skin rash, or lymphadenopathy. The reaction is believed to result from release of treponemal antigens following rapid killing of *T. pallidum*; it typically begins 6–12 h after treatment and resolves within 24 h.

Recommended Regimens

PRIMARY, SECONDARY, AND EARLY-LATENT INFECTION

Treatment of choice

- Benzathine penicillin G 2.4 million units IM, single dose

Alternative regimens for penicillin-allergic patients

- Doxycycline 100 mg PO *bid* for 2 weeks
- Tetracycline HCl 500 mg PO *qid* for 2 weeks

Treatment of HIV-infected patients

- Benzathine penicillin G 2.4 million units IM, as for persons without HIV infection; some experts recommend repeating same regimen weekly for total of 2 or 3 doses
- Only penicillin should be used; allergic patients should be desensitized and treated with penicillin

LATE SYPHILIS (>1 YEAR DURATION), EXCEPT NEUROSYPHILIS

Treatment of choice

- Benzathine penicillin G 2.4 million units IM weekly for 3 doses

Alternative regimens

- Doxycycline 100 mg orally *bid* for 4 weeks
- Tetracycline HCl 500 mg orally *qid* for 4 weeks

NEUROSYPHILIS

Treatment of choice

- Aqueous penicillin G 3 to 4 million units IV every 4 h for 10 to 14 days

Alternative regimens

- Procaine penicillin G 2.4 million units IM daily, plus probenecid 500 mg PO *qid,* for 10 to 14 days
- Only penicillin has been shown to be effective; penicillin-allergic patients should be desensitized and treated with penicillin

SYPHILIS IN PREGNANT WOMEN

Penicillin, appropriate to clinical stage; allergic patients should be desensitized and treated with penicillin; tetracyclines are contraindicated in pregnancy; erythromycin does not treat fetal infection

CONGENITAL SYPHILIS   Treatment issues are complex; treat with penicillin in consultation with an expert

Follow-up

PRIMARY, SECONDARY, AND EARLY-LATENT SYPHILIS   Reexamine and obtain quantitative VDRL or RPR 1, 3, 6, and 12 months after treatment or until negative; if VDRL or RPR remain reactive at any titer, repeat at 6- to 12-month intervals for 1–2 years

LATE SYPHILIS   Reexamine and obtain quantitative VDRL or RPR after 3, 6, and 12 months; repeat at 12-month intervals for 2–3 years if test remains reactive

HIV-INFECTED PATIENTS   Reexamine and obtain quantitative VDRL or RPR 1, 2, 3, 6, 9, 12, and 24 months after treatment; repeat at all intervals, even if test becomes negative before 24 months

NEUROSYPHILIS   Follow as appropriate for stage and HIV status; if CSF abnormal before treatment, repeat CSF examination at 6-month intervals until cell count within normal limits and CSF–VDRL tests negative

PREVENTION

Management of Sex Partners   Examine and obtain serologic tests for syphilis for all sex partners exposed during infectious period, usually from exposure to start of treatment; treat seronegative partners who have had sex with an infectious case within preceding 3 months, using benzathine penicillin or other regimen effective against early syphilis; local or state health department usually will assist in identifying and notifying partners

Screening   Routine serology for persons at risk, especially those with characteristics of core transmitters; most states require testing of all pregnant women

Reporting   Required by law in all states, to compile accurate statistics required to allocate resources, target prevention programs, and facilitate counseling and partner management services; primary, secondary, or early-latent syphilis normally should be promptly reported by telephone.

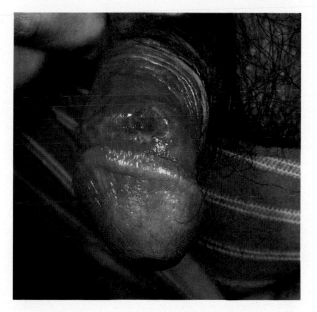

4–1. *Chancre of penis in primary syphilis.*

Patient Profile   Age 25, gay computer programmer

History   Painless sore on penis for 10 days; frequently visits a bath house, where he has sex with anonymous partners and inhales amyl nitrite ("poppers")

Examination   Indurated, nontender ulcer of penis, without purulent exudate; bilateral inguinal lymphadenopathy with 2- to 3-cm rubbery, slightly tender nodes

Differential Diagnosis   Classic chancre is highly specific for syphilis, but consider herpes and chancroid; slim possibility of cancer and other nonsexually transmitted conditions

Laboratory   Darkfield microscopy positive for *T. pallidum*; stat RPR positive; VDRL positive (titer 1:8), TPPA reactive; lesion culture for herpes simplex virus (negative); rectal and pharyngeal screening tests for *N. gonorrhoeae* and *C. trachomatis* (both negative); HIV serology, with appropriate counseling (negative)

Diagnosis   Primary syphilis

Treatment   Benzathine penicillin G 2.4 million units IM

Management of Partners   Patient interviewed by health department counselor, but no identifiable partners elicited

Comment   Classic presentation of primary syphilis; treatment would have been warranted even if darkfield and serological tests for syphilis had been negative; patient counseled about HIV risks and prevention; follow-up syphilis serology scheduled after 1, 3, 6, and 12 months

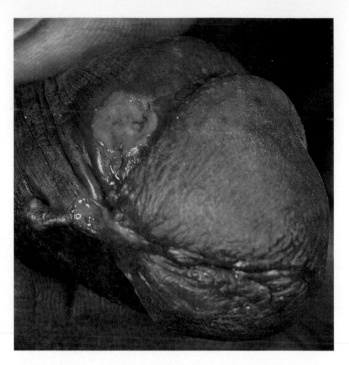

4–2. *Two penile chancres in primary syphilis.*

Patient Profile   Age 32, married assembly line worker with 4-year history of recurrent genital herpes

History   Penile sores 3 weeks; delayed seeking care because "I thought my herpes was back"; treated 5 years previously for secondary syphilis; occasional anonymous sex with other men in bars or parks

Examination   Two indurated, slightly tender penile lesions, with membranous white exudate; bilateral, shotty, nontender inguinal lymphadenopathy

Differential Diagnosis   Primary syphilis, recurrent herpes; possible chancroid

Laboratory   Darkfield examination positive for spirochetes; stat RPR positive; VDRL reactive, titer 1:64; HSV culture negative; HIV serology negative

Diagnosis   Primary syphilis

Treatment   Benzathine penicillin G 2.4 million units IM

Management of Partners   Patient referred his wife, who was found to be VDRL-negative; treated with benzathine penicillin G

Other   Presentation with two lesions and their appearance suggested possibility of genital herpes, but multiple chancres occasionally occur in syphilis; treponemal confirmatory test not indicated because positive results are probable, owing to prior secondary syphilis; scheduled for repeat HIV serology after 3 months; at patient's request, he was referred for professional counseling to address his compulsive risky sexual behavior

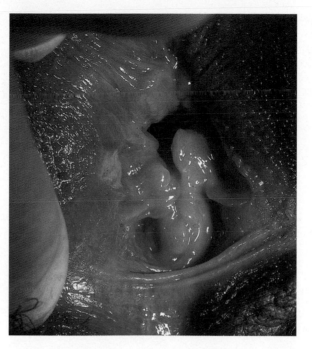

4–3. *Primary syphilis: darkfield-positive chancre; atypically tender, nonindurated lesion.*

Patient Profile Age 22, unemployed, crack cocaine addict

History Painful genital sore for 5 days; only recent sex partner was her boyfriend, who 1 month previously was released following a 6-month jail term

Examination Superficial, exquisitely tender ulcer of vestibule; no lymphadenopathy or skin rash

Differential Diagnosis Genital herpes, syphilis, chancroid, trauma; less likely considerations include Behçet's disease, Stevens-Johnson syndrome, and others

Laboratory Darkfield microscopy positive for *T. pallidum*; stat RPR, VDRL, HSV culture (all negative); tests for *N. gonorrhoeae* and *C. trachomatis* (both negative); HIV serology negative

Diagnosis Primary syphilis

Treatment Benzathine penicillin G 2.4 million units IM

Partner Management Partner referred and found to have early-latent syphilis (VDRL 1:16, documented negative during an STD clinic visit 9 months earlier); treated with benzathine penicillin G

Comment Clinical presentation suggested herpes or chancroid; some patients with primary syphilis present before developing reactive serological tests; follow-up syphilis serology testing scheduled after 1, 3, 6, and 12 months

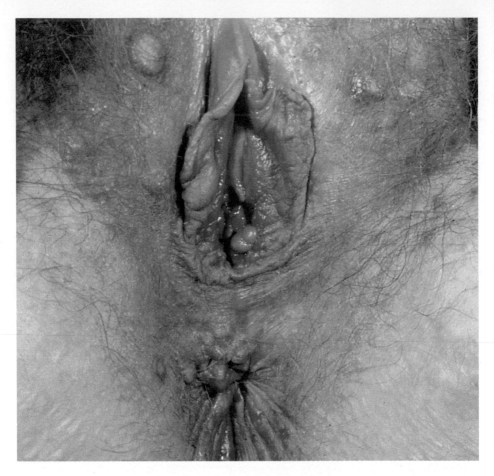

4–4. *Condylomata lata in secondary syphilis; such lesions contain large numbers of* T. pallidum *(often darkfield-positive) and are highly infectious.*

Patient Profile   Age 19, single beautician

History   Referred for consultation because of genital and perianal warts of 6 weeks' duration, not responding to repeated weekly applications of podophyllin; 3 sex partners in previous 6 months; unconfirmed history of "severe reaction" to penicillin in early childhood

Examination   Several flat, firm, slightly erythematous papular excrescences of perineum and perinatally; some perianal lesions superficially ulcerated; bilateral nontender inguinal lymphadenopathy

Differential Diagnosis   Secondary syphilis, genital warts, herpes

Laboratory   Darkfield microscopy negative; stat RPR positive; VDRL positive, titer 1:128; TPPA positive; HIV serology and cultures for HSV, *C. trachomatis,* and *N. gonorrhoeae* all negative

Diagnosis   Secondary syphilis with condylomata lata

Treatment   Doxycycline 100 mg PO *bid* for 2 weeks

Comment   All lesions resolved within 1 week; diagnosis was delayed because syphilis serology was not done in presence of presumed genital warts due to human papillomavirus; treated with doxycycline because of history of penicillin allergy; follow-up syphilis serology scheduled after 1, 3, 6, and 12 months; patient interviewed by counselor to identify and treat sex partners

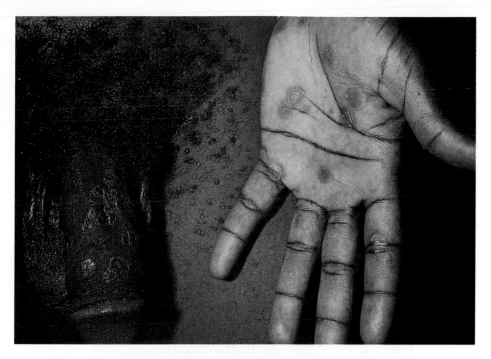

4–5. *Secondary syphilis rash of penis and palms.*

Patient Profile Age 26, unemployed, IV drug user

History Painless, nonpruritic skin rash of hands, trunk, and penis; anorexia and 10-pound weight loss over 3 months; transient painless penile sore that resolved spontaneously 2 months earlier; "several" female sex partners in past year

Examination Papulosquamous, nonpruritic eruption of genitals, trunk, extremities, palms, and soles; prominent 2- to 3-cm nontender cervical, inguinal, and supraclavicular lymph nodes

Differential Diagnosis Secondary syphilis, pityriasis rosea, viral syndrome, allergic rash, HIV infection

Laboratory Stat RPR positive; VDRL reactive, titer 1:512; MHA-TP positive; HIV serology positive

Diagnosis Secondary syphilis; HIV infection

Treatment Benzathine penicillin G 2.4 million units IM, repeated after 1 week

Management of Partners Health department counselor and patient worked together to identify, locate, examine, and treat 3 partners; one had latent syphilis, unknown duration (asymptomatic, VDRL titer 1:4); all three were HIV-negative

Comment Higher than usual VDRL titers sometimes seen in HIV-infected persons; the treating physician elected enhanced therapy with a second dose of benzathine penicillin G due to HIV infection; patient referred for HIV evaluation and treatment; follow-up syphilis serology scheduled after 1, 2, 3, 6, 9, 12, and 24 months

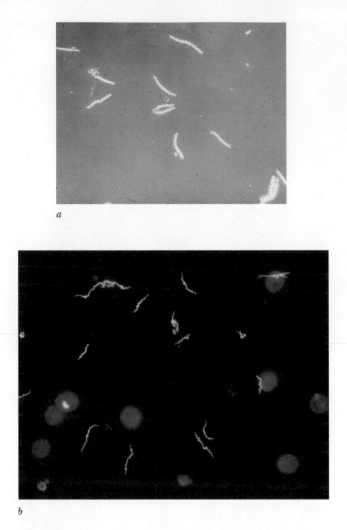

a

b

4–6. Treponema pallidum. a. *Viewed by darkfield microscopy.* b. *Stained with fluorescein-conjugated monoclonal antibody to* T. pallidum, *with red counterstain, viewed under ultraviolet light. (Courtesy of Sheila A. Lukehart, Ph.D.)*

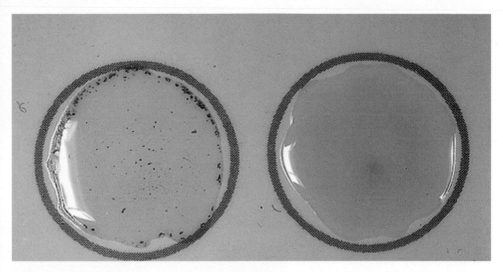

4–7. *Rapid plasma reagin (RPR) card test. Reactive serum (left) shows agglutination of carbon particles; control specimen (right) shows no agglutination. The RPR card test requires 10 minutes to perform. (Enlarged view.)*

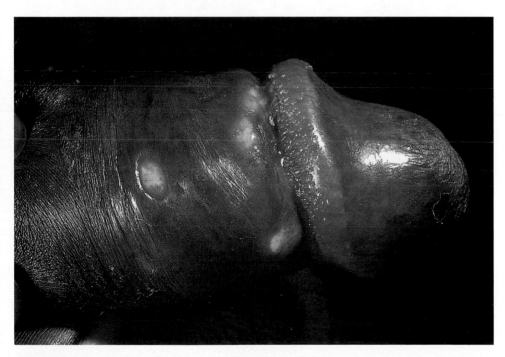

4–8. *Primary syphilis: multiple chancres of the penis, under the retracted foreskin. Multiple chancres occasionally occur, perhaps with increased frequency in moist areas such as the preputial sac.*

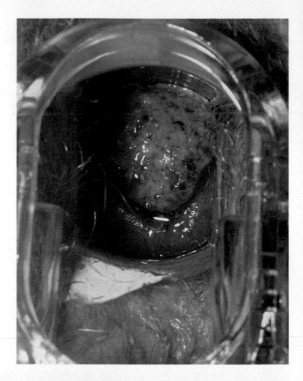

4–9. *Primary syphilis: atypical hypertrophic chancre of cervix. The patient presented with a complaint of post-coital bleeding and was initially thought to have cervical carcinoma, but syphilis was confirmed by dark-field examination, serology, and rapid resolution of the lesion following benzathine penicillin G.*

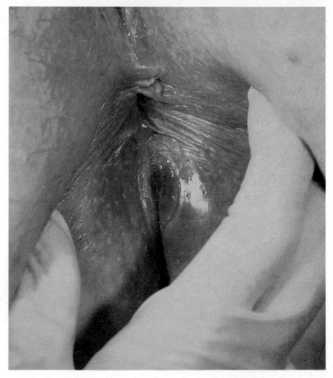

4–10. *Primary syphilis: darkfield-positive perianal chancre.*

2 BACTERIAL SEXUALLY TRANSMITTED DISEASES

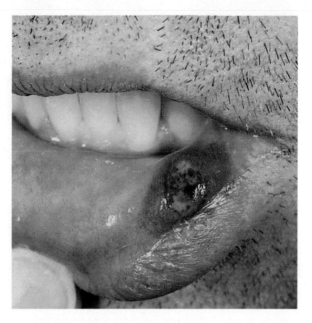

4–11. *Primary syphilis: chancre of lower lip. Although less common than genital or perianal lesions, oral chancres are not rare.*

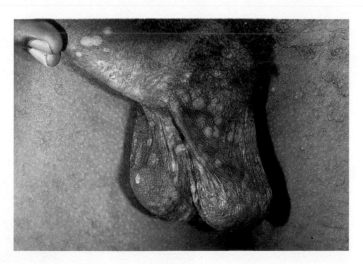

4–12. *Secondary syphilis: papular eruption of penis and scrotum. Depigmented lesions are common in dark-skinned persons.*

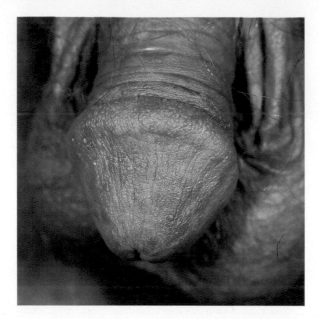

4–13. *Secondary syphilis: papulosquamous rash of penis. Note similarity to scabies (Fig. 13–2) and psoriasis (Figs. 21–3 and 21–4).*

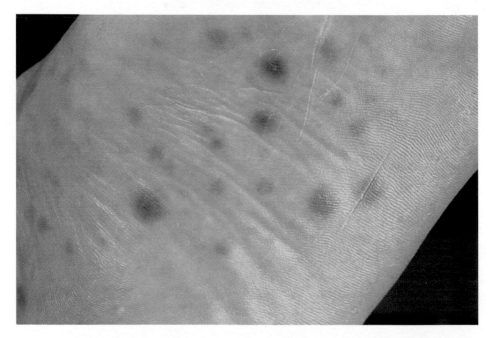

4–14. *Secondary syphilis: papular rash involving the sole of the foot.*

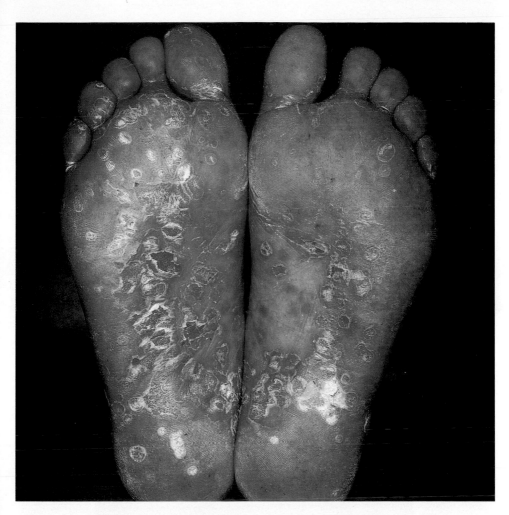

4–15. *Secondary syphilis: extensive hyperkeratotic plantar rash in an HIV-seropositive man with secondary syphilis. Note similarity to keratoderma blennorrhagica of Reiter's syndrome (Fig. 16–3).*

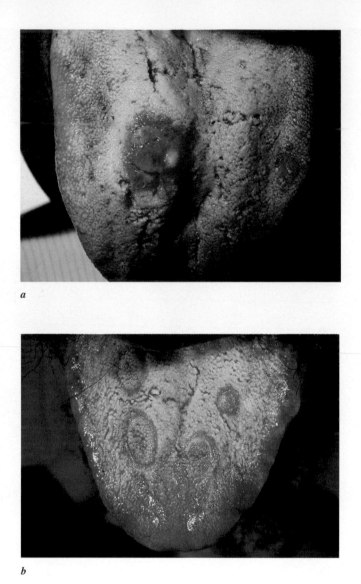

a

b

4–16. *Secondary syphilis with mucous patches of the tongue. Mucous patches can involve the oral, genital, or rectal mucous membranes; they are nontender, usually asymptomatic, and highly infectious. a. Single darkfield-positive mucous patch; although darkfield examination is often discouraged for oral lesions, it may be useful if strongly positive. b. Multiple mucous patches as well as "coated" tongue in an HIV-infected person with secondary syphilis. (From KK Holmes et al.* Sexually Transmitted Diseases, *3d ed. New York: McGraw-Hill, 1999.)*

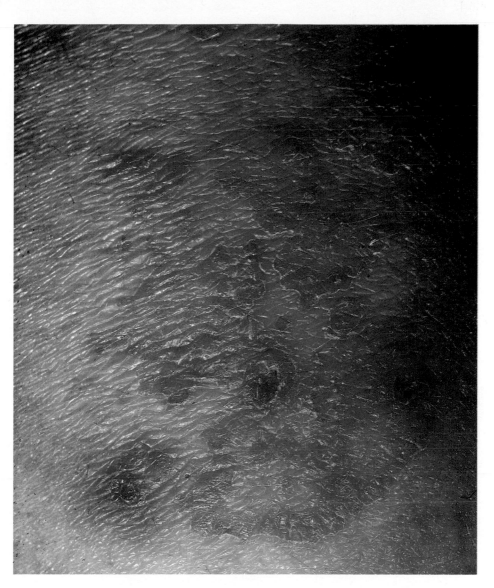

4–17.   *Secondary syphilis: atypical eczema-like rash of buttock. Despite its dry appearance, this lesion was darkfield-positive and resolved promptly after treatment with benzathine penicillin G.*

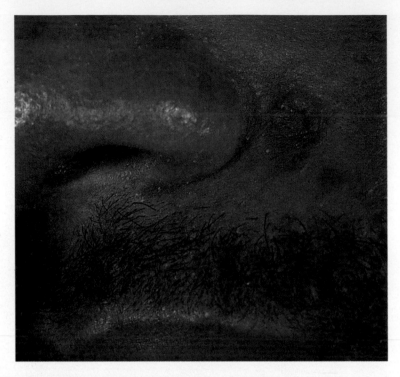

4–18. *Secondary syphilis: hyperpigmented papules of the nose and nasolabial fold. Such lesions are also commonly seen at the corners of the mouth, where they often ulcerate; such lesions are then called "split papules."*

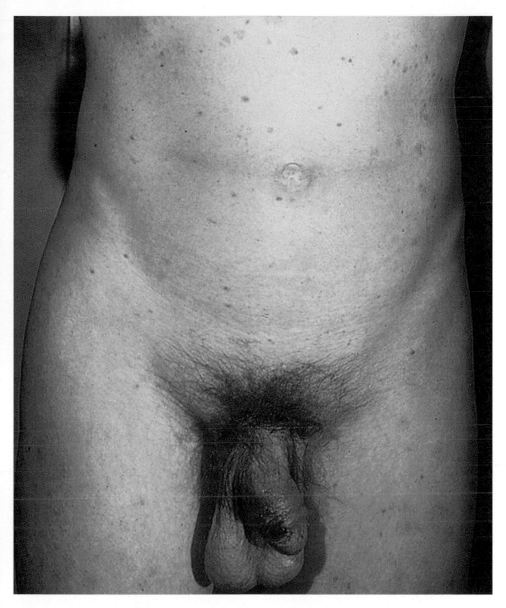

4–19. *Secondary syphilis: papulosquamous rash involving trunk and extremities. This HIV-infected patient also had a large necrotic penile ulcer (Fig. 21–11) with streptococcal cellulitis, possibly the result of secondary infection of the original chancre. Before the penile infection supervened, the patient's physician was unaware that the patient continued to be sexually active with multiple anonymous partners, and the physician failed to perform a syphilis serology, believing the rash was due to allergy to antiretroviral drugs.*

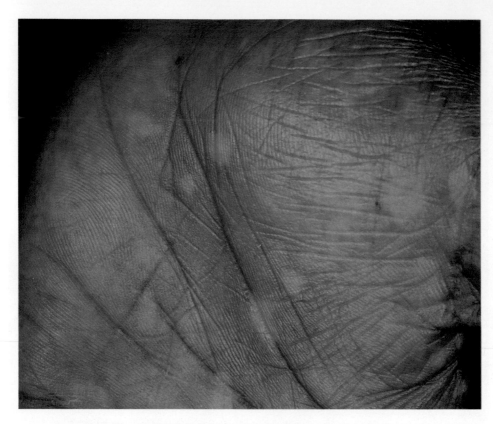

4–20. *Secondary syphilis: hypopigmented macules of palm.*

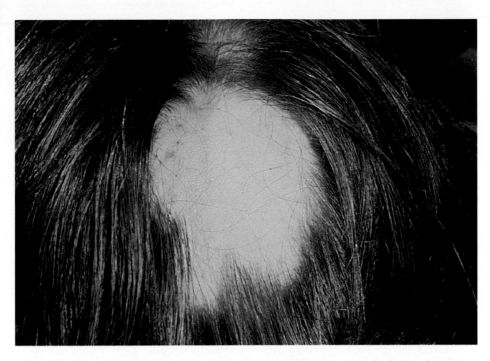

4–21. *Secondary syphilis: alopecia of scalp, mimicking alopecia areata. Syphilitic alopecia more often is patchy and irregular ("moth-eaten"). The patient had several other areas of hair loss, and regrowth began promptly following treatment for syphilis.*

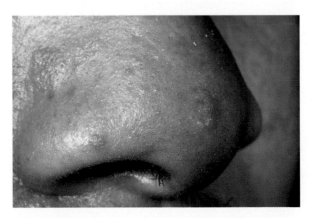

4–22. *Secondary syphilis: cutaneous nodules of nose; the nodules resolved promptly following penicillin therapy.*

ADDITIONAL READING

DiCarlo RP, Martin DH: The clinical diagnosis of genital ulcer disease in men. *Clin Infect Dis* 25:292–298, 1997. *Study of 446 men with genital ulcers, showing poor association between clinical presentation and laboratory-documented diagnosis, except that typical chancres almost always were syphilitic.*

Handsfield HH: Genital herpes, syphilis, and genital ulcer disease, in *Clinical Infectious Diseases: A Practice Approach*, RR Root et al (eds). New York, Oxford University Press, 1999: Chap 70. *A succinct, clinically oriented overview.*

Hook EW III, Marra CM: Acquired syphilis in adults. *N Engl J Med* 326:1060–1069, 1992. *A comprehensive review of the epidemiology and clinical aspects of syphilis, including interactions between syphilis and HIV infection.*

Rolfs RT et al: A randomized trial of enhanced therapy for early syphilis in patients with and without human immunodeficiency virus infection. *N Engl J Med* 337:307–314, 1997. *A study of treatment options and overview of issues related to syphilis-HIV interactions.*

Romanowski B et al: Serologic response to treatment of infectious syphilis. *Ann Intern Med* 114:1005–1009, 1991. *A study confirming older data showing high rates of reversion of treponemal serologic tests to negative following repetitive treatment of early syphilis.*

St. Louis ME, Wasserheit JN: Elimination of syphilis in the United States. *Science* 281:353–354, 1998. *Summary of potential approaches and Centers for Disease Control and Prevention's plan to achieve elimination of endogenous syphilis in the United States.*

Chapter 5
CHANCROID

Chancroid is a genital ulcer disease caused by *Haemophilus ducreyi*. It is one of the original five "classic" STDs, along with gonorrhea, syphilis, lymphogranuloma venereum, and granuloma inguinale. In most societies, chancroid is more closely linked with commercial sex or illicit drug use than are other STDs. This may be explained by the relative infrequency of an asymptomatic carrier state; maintenance of a chancroid outbreak may require a population of persons who have intercourse despite painful genital ulcers. Chancroid, like other ulcerative and inflammatory STDs, markedly enhances the efficiency of sexual transmission and acquisition of HIV. At present, chancroid is uncommon in the United States; it typically occurs in discrete outbreaks rather than as an endemic disease.

EPIDEMIOLOGY

Incidence and Prevalence Declining incidence during 1990s; 3,476 reported cases in 1991, 189 cases in 1998

Transmission Exclusively by sexual contact

Age All ages susceptible; most cases occur in patients aged 25 to 35 years

Sex No particular predilection, but diagnosed more frequently in men than women

Sexual Orientation No special predilection known; few cases reported in exclusively homosexual men or women

Other Risk Factors Intact foreskin enhances risk in men

HISTORY

Incubation Period Usually 2–10 days

Symptoms Painful ulceration is typical, sometimes with multiple lesions; about 50% of patients have painful regional (usually inguinal) lymphadenopathy; usually no systemic symptoms

Epidemiologic History Often commercial sex, illicit drug use, or recent travel to an endemic area

PHYSICAL EXAMINATION

One or more nonindurated genital ulcers with purulent bases; most common sites in men are glans, corona, or inner surface of foreskin; in women, most lesions are at introitus or labia, sometimes intravaginal; ulcers usually very tender, but nontender lesions sometimes present; surrounding erythema and undermined edges are common; multiple ulcers sometimes form "kissing" lesions due to apposition of initial lesion to uninvolved skin or mucosal surface; unilateral or bilateral inguinal lymphadenopathy in 50-60%; lymphadenopathy is characteristic of pyogenic infection, with overlying erythema, tenderness, often fluctuant; involved nodes sometimes rupture, with purulent discharge

LABORATORY DIAGNOSIS

Isolation of *H. ducreyi* from lesion or lymph node aspirate; sensitivity of culture 60–80%, depending on specimen management, variations in media, and laboratory's experience; PCR test available in some research settings, with improved sensitivity compared to culture; Gram stain of lymph node aspirate may show small gram-negative bacilli, but is insensitive and nonspecific; all suspected cases require darkfield microscopic examination, culture for HSV, and serological test for syphilis

DIAGNOSTIC CRITERIA

Identification of *H. ducreyi* by culture or PCR is definitive; otherwise, diagnosis is based on clinical findings and epidemiologic setting and exclusion of genital herpes and syphilis

TREATMENT

Principles Many strains of *H. ducreyi* contain β-lactamase plasmids, conferring resistance to penicillins; third-generation cephalosporins, fluoroquinolones (e.g., ciprofloxacin), and macrolides remain active; all therapies, especially recommended cephalosporin or fluoroquinolone regimens, less effective in HIV-infected persons

Recommended Treatments
• Azithromycin 1.0 g PO (single dose)
• ceftriaxone 250 mg IM (single dose)
• ciprofloxacin 500 mg PO bid for 3 days
• erythromycin base 500 mg PO qid for 7 days

CONTROL MEASURES

Assure referral and treatment of sex partners; appropriate diagnostic testing in selected patients with genital ulcer disease; immediately telephone report of new case to local or state health department

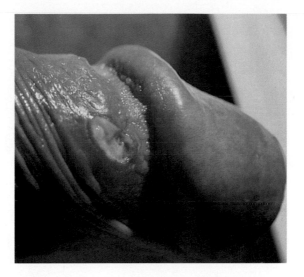

5–1. *Chancoidal ulcer of penis.*

Patient Profile   Age 26, unmarried salesman

History   Painful sore on penis for 5 days; commercial sexual exposure 10 days earlier in a country where chancroid is endemic

Examination   Tender, nonindurated ulcerative penile lesion with purulent base; uncircumcised; no lymphadenopathy

Differential Diagnosis   Genital herpes, chancroid, syphilis

Laboratory   Stat RPR and darkfield microscopy negative; culture of lesion positive for *H. ducreyi*, negative for HSV; urethral tests for *N. gonorrhoeae* and *C. trachomatis* negative; HIV serology negative

Diagnosis   Chancroid

Treatment   Azithromycin 1.0 g PO, single dose

Comment   Lesion healed within 7 days; current girlfriend had normal examination, with negative vaginal culture for *H. ducreyi*, treated with azithromycin; patient scheduled for follow-up VDRL after 1 month and repeat HIV serology after 3 months

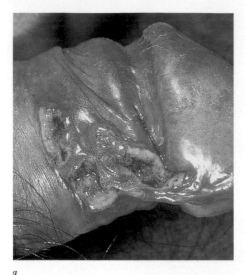

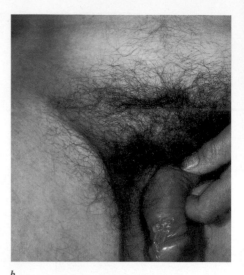

a

b

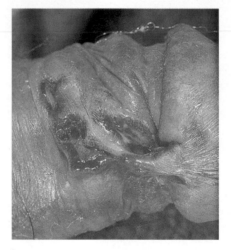

c

5–2. *Chancroid. a. Penile ulcers under foreskin; the ulceration had perforated the frenulum of the penis, through which a probe could be passed. b. Inguinal swelling and erythema. c. Healing ulcers 1 week after starting treatment; reduced purulent exudate and partial reepithelialization.*

Patient Profile Age 60, married, businessman with a large international corporation

History Painful, enlarging penile ulcers for 2 weeks; onset 5 days after sexual exposure in Africa; painful right inguinal swelling for 3 days; company's occupational medicine clinic treated patient with amoxicillin, without improvement after 5 days

Examination Multiple, coalescing, irregularly shaped, purulent tender ulcers under foreskin; 3× 5-cm indurated, tender, nonfluctuant right inguinal lymph node; inguinal erythema extending to the low abdominal wall

Differential Diagnosis Classic chancroid; rule out herpes, syphilis; LGV unlikely; possible secondary pyogenic infection

Laboratory *H. ducreyi* isolated by culture; darkfield examination, VDRL, culture for HSV (all negative); urethral cultures for *N. gonorrhoeae* and *C. trachomatis* (negative); HIV serology (negative)

Diagnosis Chancroid

Treatment Ceftriaxone 250 mg IM, single dose, followed by amoxicillin with clavulanic acid (Augmentin) 500/125 mg PO *tid* for 10 days

Management of Sex Partner (s) Patient advised to notify his partner in Africa; had not resumed intercourse with his wife

Comment Amoxicillin/clavulanic acid was prescribed because the atypically extensive inguinal erythema suggested secondary pyogenic cellulitis; the ulcers healed rapidly and erythema regressed, but lymph node gradually became fluctuant and required a needle aspiration 10 days after start of treatment. Follow-up VDRL was negative after 1 month, and repeat HIV serology was negative after 1 and 3 months. At numerous visits to his company's occupational medicine clinic in anticipation of international travel, the patient—who regularly was sexually active with local residents when traveling—was routinely offered appropriate immunizations, malaria prophylaxis, and advice to avoid food-borne illness, but was never asked about plans for sexual activity or advised about condoms or other aspects of safer sex. Some persons view travel as an opportunity for sexual adventure, and clinicians should include advice about STD prevention when counseling travelers.

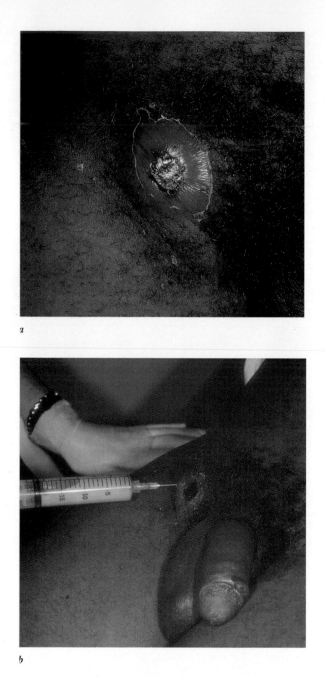

a

b

5–3. *Chancroid. a. Fluctuant lymph node, with eschar that followed spontaneous rupture with partial drainage. b. Needle aspiration of lymph node; the penile ulcer also is visible.*

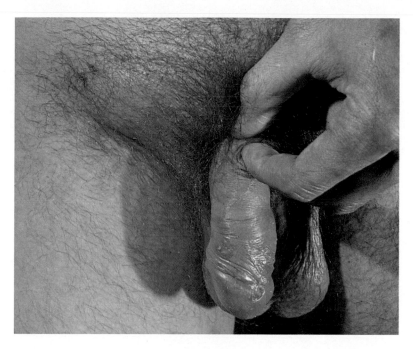

5–4. *Chancroid, with penile ulcers and prominent inguinal lymphadenopathy with overlying erythema. The small eschars lateral to the lymph node mark the sites of previous needle aspirations.*

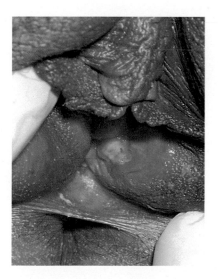

5–5. *Chancroidal ulcer of vaginal introitus. (Reproduced with permission from KK Holmes et al.* Sexually Transmitted Diseases, *3d ed. New York: McGraw-Hill, 1999.)*

ADDITIONAL READING

DiCarlo RP et al: Chancroid epidemiology in New Orleans men. *J Infect Dis* 172:446–452, 1995. *Description of a large outbreak, illustrating clinical and epidemiologic features of chancroid that apply to most outbreaks in the United States.*

Morse SA et al: Comparison of clinical diagnosis and standard laboratory and molecular methods for the diagnosis of genital ulcer disease in Lesotho: association with human immunodeficiency virus infection. *J Infect Dis* 175:583–589, 1997. *Documentation of the superiority of PCR over traditional methods to diagnose chancroid, syphilis, and genital herpes.*

Ronald AR, Albritton W: Chancroid and *Haemophilus ducreyi,* in *Sexually Transmitted Diseases,* 3d ed, KK Holmes et al (eds). New York, McGraw-Hill, 1999, Chap 38. *A comprehensive review in the definitive textbook on STDs*

Schmid GP: Treatment of chancroid, 1997. *Clin Infect Dis* 28(Suppl 1):S14–S20, 1999. *Review of treatment issues for chancroid, as background for CDC's 1998 STD Treatment Guidelines.*

Chapter 6
GRANULOMA INGUINALE (DONOVANOSIS)

Granuloma inguinale, or donovanosis, is a genital ulcer disease that is rare even in most developing countries. Endemic foci exist in the Indian subcontinent, Papua New Guinea, and parts of Brazil, Australia, and central and southern Africa. The causative organism, *Calymmatobacterium granulomatis,* is a Gram-negative bacillus closely related to *Klebsiella* species; it was recently proposed that the nomenclature be revised to *Klebsiella granulomatis. C. granulomatis* was only recently grown in sustained culture; it is hoped that improved diagnostic tests and understanding of pathogenesis will soon follow. The disease may be highly destructive, but is more often indolent, progressing slowly for several years. There is rare systemic dissemination, usually manifested by hepatic and osteolytic lesions. Granuloma inguinale sometimes causes cervical lymphadenitis in infants (typically <6 months old), presumably the result of perinatal exposure. The response to antimicrobial therapy is said to be slower in HIV-infected patients.

EPIDEMIOLOGY

Incidence and Prevalence Rare in the United States (most cases probably imported from other countries); 0 to 10 cases reported annually from 1995 to 1998

Transmission Primarily by sexual contact, but location of some nongenital lesions suggest some cases transmitted by nonsexual routes; some sex partners of chronically infected patients remain free of disease for several years; perinatal transmission to newborns

Age No specific predilection known; most patients aged 20 to 40 years

Sex Male:female case ratios vary from 1:1 to 6:1 in endemic areas, perhaps related to exposure patterns (e.g., commercial sex)

Sexual Orientation No known predisposition; few cases reported in homosexual men or women

HISTORY

Incubation Period Usually 2 weeks to 3 months

Symptoms Indolent genital ulcer, often painless; sometimes multiple lesions; chronic cases may be very extensive; occasional inguinal swelling; usually no systemic symptoms

Epidemiologic History In the United States, sexual exposure in an endemic area is the dominant risk factor

PHYSICAL EXAMINATION

Four clinical variants described: ulcerogranulomatous, with hypertrophic, red granulation tissue and readily induced bleeding; hypertrophic, manifesting exuberant exophytic wartlike ("verruciform") lesions; necrotic, with deep ulcers and extensive tissue destruction; and sclerotic, with extensive fibrosis, sometimes with urethral stricture; usually no overtly purulent exudate; may mimic carcinoma; usually involves penis or vulva, sometimes perianal, rarely nongenital sites; lymphadenopathy absent, but "pseudobubo" results from subcutaneous extension of inflammatory tissue, with inguinal mass; rarely extensive ulceration lasting several years, sometimes resulting in autoamputation of penis; rare osseous dissemination, with hepatic or osteolytic lesions; cervical lymphadenitis in children <6 months old

LABORATORY DIAGNOSIS

Histologic identification of organism in vacuoles within macrophages ("Donovan bodies") in biopsied tissue or crush preparation (using modified Giemsa stain); an experimental PCR assay has been described

DIAGNOSTIC CRITERIA

Clinical appearance, plus biopsy or crush preparation showing characteristic histopathology; exposure history; exclusion of other causes

TREATMENT

Principles   Antimicrobial susceptibility surmised primarily by clinical response to various drugs; all regimens administered for at least 3 weeks, or until healing complete (up to 3 months)

Treatments of Choice

- Trimethoprim/sulfamethoxazole 800/160 mg (one double-strength tablet) PO *bid*

- Doxycycline 100 mg PO *bid*

Alternative Regimens   Ciprofloxacin 750 mg PO *bid*;

- Erythromycin base 500 mg PO qid;

- Azithromycin 500 mg PO daily for 7 days, or 1.0 g PO weekly for 4 weeks

PREVENTION AND CONTROL

Identifiable sex partners should be treated; condoms probably provide partial protection

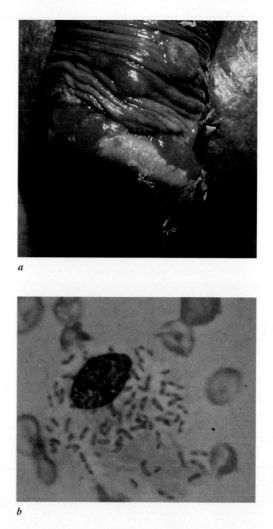

a

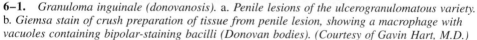

b

6–1. *Granuloma inguinale (donovanosis). a. Penile lesions of the ulcerogranulomatous variety. b. Giemsa stain of crush preparation of tissue from penile lesion, showing a macrophage with vacuoles containing bipolar-staining bacilli (Donovan bodies). (Courtesy of Gavin Hart, M.D.)*

Patient Profile Age 47, merchant seaman

History Painless penile sores for 3 weeks; during 2 months prior to onset had intercourse with commercial sex workers in several ports, including coastal cities in India

Examination Multiple, slightly tender, hypertrophic ulcerative penile lesions; no lymphadenopathy

Differential Diagnosis Granuloma inguinale (donovanosis), primary syphilis, squamous cell cancer

Laboratory Giemsa stain of crush preparation of biopsy specimen showed large mononuclear cells with Donovan bodies; darkfield examination, lesion cultures for HSV and *Haemophilus ducreyi*, VDRL, HIV serology (all negative)

Diagnosis Granuloma inguinale

Treatment Doxycycline 100 mg PO *bid* for 3 weeks

Partner Management No domestic partners; foreign partners unidentified

Follow-up Lesions regressed and were partly re-epithelialized after 10 days; patient then lost to further follow-up

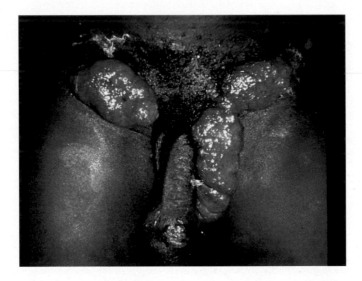

6–2. *Granuloma inguinale. Extensive hypertrophic granulomatous lesions. (Reproduced with permission from KK Holmes et al,* Sexually Transmitted Diseases, *3d ed. New York, McGraw-Hill, 1999.)*

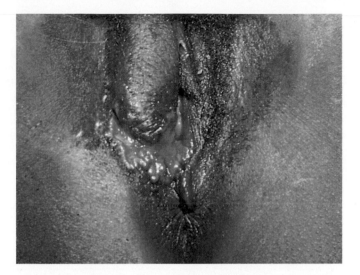

6–3. *Granuloma inguinale with extensive genital ulceration and vulvar lymphedema.* *(Reproduced with permission from KK Holmes et al,* Sexually Transmitted Diseases, *3d ed. New York, McGraw-Hill, 1999.)*

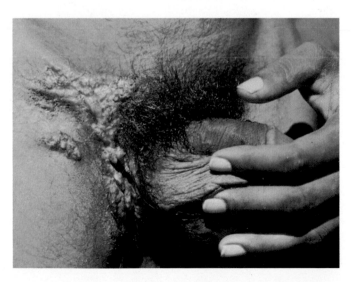

6–4. *Granuloma inguinale with hypertrophic verruciform lesions. (Reproduced with permission from KK Holmes et al,* Sexually Transmitted Diseases, *3d ed. New York, McGraw-Hill, 1999.)*

ADDITIONAL READING

Association of Genitourinary Medicine and Medical Society for Study of Venereal Diseases: National guideline for the management of donovanosis (granuloma inguinale). *Sex Transm Infect* 75 (suppl 1): S38–S39, 1999. *Summary of diagnosis and treatment recommendations in the United Kingdom.*

Jamkhedkar PP et al: Clinico-epidemiologic features of granuloma inguinale in the era of acquired immune deficiency syndrome. *Sex Transm Dis* 25:196–200, 1998. *Comparison of the natural course and response to treatment, showing increased tissue destruction and delayed therapeutic response in HIV-infected compared with HIV-negative patients.*

O'Farrell N: Donovanosis, in *Sexually Transmitted Diseases*, KK Holmes et al (eds). New York, McGraw-Hill, 1999, Chap 39. *A comprehensive review by the leading authority on donovanosis.*

VIRAL SEXUALLY TRANSMITTED DISEASES

Chapter 7
GENITAL HERPES

Genital herpes is the most common cause of genital ulceration in industrialized countries, with an estimated annual incidence of one million cases and a prevalence of 50 to 60 million persons in the United States. Most cases are caused by herpes simplex virus type 2 (HSV-2), but many are due to HSV type 1 (HSV-1), the usual cause of orolabial herpes. Infection with either HSV type is life-long; the virus persists in neural tissue, typically in the dorsal nerve root ganglia. The presence of specific antibody denotes current infection and the potential for clinical recurrences, subclinical viral shedding, and transmission of the virus to sex partners.

Most cases of genital herpes are subclinical, although most apparently asymptomatic infected persons have mild or nonspecific clinical manifestations that are ignored or whose significance is not understood by the infected person, his or her clinician, or both. Healing of lesions is accelerated and recurrent outbreaks can be prevented by systemic treatment with antiviral drugs, but no cure exists. Treatment reduces subclinical viral shedding but does not entirely eliminate it, and the efficacy of treatment in preventing transmission from subclinical infection is not yet known. The most serious complication of genital herpes is neonatal infection, acquired perinatally, which often is fatal or causes permanent neurodevelopmental sequelae. Genital herpes, like all inflammatory STDs, is associated with enhanced transmission of HIV.

EPIDEMIOLOGY

Incidence and Prevalence National seroprevalence of HSV-2 antibody 17% in 1978, rising to 22% in 1991 (+30%); at least 45 million persons in the United States now infected with HSV-2, plus several million with genital HSV-1 infection; estimated annual physician visits for first-episode genital herpes rose from about 100,000 in 1970s to about 200,000 in mid-1990s, reflecting rising incidence, increased patient concern, and improved diagnosis

Transmission Only by direct contact with infected lesions or secretions; most transmission probably results from subclinical infection; transmitted perinatally to infants, especially in presence of initial maternal genital herpes; rare autoinoculation or nosocomial infection (e.g., herpetic whitlow, keratoconjunctivitis)

Age All ages susceptible; highest acquisition rates in age range 25–35

Sex Women more susceptible than men, probably owing to larger surface area exposed; national seroprevalence of HSV-2 in 1991: 25% in women, 18% in men

Sexual Orientation Men who have sex with men (MSM) have particularly high HSV-2 seroprevalence

Other Risk Factors HSV-2 seroprevalence substantially higher in lower-income socioeconomic populations and in the southeast United States

CLINICAL CLASSIFICATION

Primary Herpes First infection with either HSV-1 or HSV-2; patient seronegative for both types at onset; symptomatic cases commonly severe, often prolonged (2–3 weeks); mucosal involvement, regional lymphadenopathy, regional neuropathy, and systemic manifestations common; 20–40% of cases due to HSV-1, acquired by either genital or orogenital exposure

Initial Nonprimary Herpes First clinical episode in presence of existing antibody, to opposite HSV type; most cases due to HSV-2 in persons seropositive for HSV-1; systemic manifestations uncommon; 40% of apparent initial cases are first-recognized recurrence in persons with longstanding infection

Recurrent Herpes Second or subsequent symptomatic outbreak due to same virus type; most cases clinically mild; lymphadenopathy, neuropathy, and systemic manifestations uncommon; because HSV-1 causes few clinical recurrences, HSV-2 is cause of >90% of recurrent genital herpes

Subclinical Infection Most cases of HSV infection, whether primary, nonprimary initial, or recurrent, are subclinical; includes truly asymptomatic and symptomatic but unrecognized infection; occurs in both never-symptomatic patients and between recognized clinical recurrences; subclinical shedding can be detected by culture 2–7% of asymptomatic days in first year after symptomatic initial genital herpes, and 1–3% of days thereafter (higher if polymerase chain reaction [PCR] assay used instead of culture)

HISTORY

Incubation Period Usually 2–10 days for symptomatic initial herpes, occasionally up to 3 weeks

Symptoms

PRIMARY HERPES Multiple genital or perianal lesions, usually bilateral or midline; many women have erosive cervicitis; painful urethritis common in men; cutaneous lesions evolve over 7–15 days from papule, to vesicle, to pustule, to ulcer, to crust; mucosal and moist lesions (e.g., vulva, urethra, under foreskin) ulcerate early, often with severe pain; repeated crops of lesions may appear over 3–6 weeks; frequent inguinal pain and swelling, dysuria, and vaginal or urethral discharge; often neuropathic symptoms referable to sacral nerve roots (e.g., urinary retention, constipation, paresthesias); fever, malaise, headache often present; occasionally photophobia, stiff neck

FIRST EPISODE NONPRIMARY HERPES Usually fewer lesions than primary herpes; untreated duration typically 10–14 days; inguinal pain and swelling less common than in primary infection; discharge, dysuria, and systemic and neuropathic symptoms uncommon

RECURRENT HERPES Usually few lesions, lateralized to one side of midline; >90% of patients with symptomatic initial HSV-2 infection have symptomatic recurrences; in first year after initial infection with HSV-2, mean 5 outbreaks annually in men, 4 in women; 40% of patients have ≥6 and 20% have ≥10 outbreaks per year; symptomatic recurrences substantially less common in genital HSV-1 infection; repeated symptomatic outbreaks usually involve same area of penis, vulva, anus, or buttocks; some patients have prodrome of paresthesias 1–2 days before lesions; evolution through papular, vesicular, pustular, ulcerative, and crust stages more rapid than in initial herpes, usually 7–10 days; atypical ulcerative lesions common; inguinal swelling and systemic symptoms rare; neuropathic symptoms rare (except prodrome); debilitating, erosive ulcers common in persons with HIV or other immunodeficiency; rare CNS reactivation of HSV-2 causes recurrent aseptic (Mollaret's) meningitis

Epidemiologic History High prevalence in all population subgroups; many patients lack typical high-risk STD profiles; history of exposure to infected sex partner or new partner often diagnostically helpful, but often absent

PHYSICAL EXAMINATION

Erythematous papules, vesicles, pustules, ulcers, or crusts; lesions often occur in clusters; individual lesions typically 2–5 mm diameter, but all sizes and shapes occur; ulcers usually tender, nonindurated; many lesions small, "nonspecific" in appearance; lymphadenopathy, when present, usually is bilateral, firm, moderately tender, without fluctuance or cutaneous erythema; erosive cervicitis or urethritis (often with localized tenderness along penile shaft) is common in primary infection; occasional sacral nerve neurological deficits (e.g., hypotonic bladder, lax anal sphincter); deeply erosive genital, perianal, or perioral lesions common in AIDS patients; nuchal rigidity and photophobia sometimes present; erythema multiforme sometimes occurs as systemic response to recurrent genital herpes

LABORATORY DIAGNOSIS

Virus Isolation Isolation in cell culture is test of choice to identify HSV in lesions; yield highest in initial episodes or from recurrent lesions <2 days old; recommended in workup of all patients with genital ulcer disease

Other Direct Tests PCR assay for HSV DNA available in some laboratories and more sensitive than culture, but not commercially available; direct-fluorescence microscopy and other immunochemical tests for HSV may approach sensitivity of culture in samples from fresh genital lesions, but most assays do not distinguish HSV-2 from HSV-1; cytologic methods (Tzanck test with Giemsa or Papanicolaou stain) insensitive, rarely indicated

Serology Noncommercial Western blot assay remains serological gold standard; accurate type-specific HSV-2 antibody tests recently became commercially available; most previous tests (e.g., indirect fluorescent antibody, neutralization assay) did not distinguish HSV-1 from HSV-2 antibody, despite claims to the contrary, and have little or no role in diagnosing or screening for genital herpes

DIAGNOSTIC CRITERIA

Clinical diagnosis often reliable in typical cases (e.g., clustered vesicles); virologic diagnosis recommended for all suspected cases; identification of HSV in lesion by culture, PCR, or immunochemical method is definitive, but negative result does not exclude herpes; positive type-specific HSV-2 antibody test often useful for patients with atypical or culture-negative lesions; rule out syphilis, chancroid, and other causes of genital ulcer by appropriate laboratory tests

TREATMENT

Antiviral Chemotherapy Systemic acyclovir, valacyclovir, or famciclovir is mainstay of therapy; valacyclovir and famciclovir offer improved bioavailability compared with acylovir; manufacturer recommends administering acyclovir 5 times daily, but pharmacokinetics and clinical experience support less frequent dosing (*tid* or *bid*); treatment speeds clinical resolution, prevents clinical recurrences, and reduces subclinical viral shedding, but does not eradicate HSV; no evidence exists for increased severity or frequency of recurrent outbreaks ("rebound effect") after suppressive treatment; effect of treatment on transmission to sex partners unknown; topical therapy has little clinical effect, rarely indicated

INITIAL (PRIMARY AND NONPRIMARY) GENITAL HERPES All cases should be treated, even if apparently mild, to shorten duration of symptoms and prevent accelerated course

- Valacyclovir 1.0 g PO *bid* for 7–10 days
- Famciclovir 250 mg PO *tid* for 7–10 days
- Acyclovir 400 mg PO *tid* for 7–10 days
- Severe cases requiring hospitalization: Acyclovir 5–10 mg/kg body weight IV every 8 h for 5–7 days or until improved, then change to oral valacyclovir, famciclovir, or acyclovir to complete 7–14 days total therapy

RECURRENT GENITAL HERPES Episodic therapy speeds healing of recurrent outbreaks if started within 1 day of onset; patients with prodrome may abort outbreaks by prompt treatment; suppressive therapy reduces symptomatic recurrences by 70–80%; suppressive therapy should be offered to all patients with recurrent herpes, especially if severe, if there is significant stress, anxiety, or depression due to recurrent herpes, or if patient has ≥6 recurrences per year; after suppression achieved, adjust regimen to determine optimal dose and frequency; discontinue suppressive therapy at 1-year intervals to reassess frequency and severity of outbreaks; effect of therapy on transmission to sex partners is unknown

Regimens for Episodic Treatment

- Valacyclovir 500 mg PO bid for 5 days
- Famciclovir 125 mg PO bid for 5 days
- Acyclovir 400 mg PO bid for 5 days

Regimens for Suppressive Treatment

- Valacyclovir 500 mg PO daily; or 1.0 g PO daily for patients with $10 symptomatic outbreaks per year
- Famciclovir 250 mg PO bid
- Acyclovir 400 mg PO bid

Supportive Therapy Keep lesions clean and dry by washing 2–3 times daily and wearing loosely fitting cotton underwear; topical anesthetic ointment may help control pain

Counseling Counsel patient about likelihood of recurrences, frequency of subclinical shedding (especially in first 6–12 months following initial infection), and potential for transmission; advise that cesarean delivery usually not necessary for women with recurrent herpes; inform patients that effective drugs are available to prevent or treat future recurrences; advise condoms to prevent transmission, especially in first year following initial infection

PREVENTION

Management of Sex Partners Evaluate all partners not known to have genital herpes; type-specific serology routinely indicated for partners to diagnose subclinical infection and aid counseling; educate patients and partners to understand subclinical infection and recognize subtle symptoms; promptly (within 24–48 h) examine partners if or when such symptoms appear or recur; reassure patient and partners that if transmission occurs, infection may cause few or no symptoms, and effective therapy available if symptoms occur

Screening Patients who request comprehensive evaluation for common STDs should be offered type-specific HSV serological testing; however, if patient at low risk (likelihood of infection <20%), false-positive results may be common and confirmatory test (e.g., Western blot at a reference laboratory) may be required

Prevention of Neonatal Herpes Highest risk of transmission follows first episode of maternal genital HSV infection in third trimester; serological testing of pregnant women and, if seronegative, their sex partners may help prevent neonatal herpes by identifying discordant couples and counseling them to avoid intercourse or orogenital exposure (depending on infected partner's HSV type) in third trimester; cesarean section indicated for women with overt herpes lesions at term; in women with symptomatic recurrent herpes, prophylactic acyclovir near term may prevent otherwise unnecessary cesarean deliveries; routine tests to detect subclinical HSV shedding not indicated in pregnant women

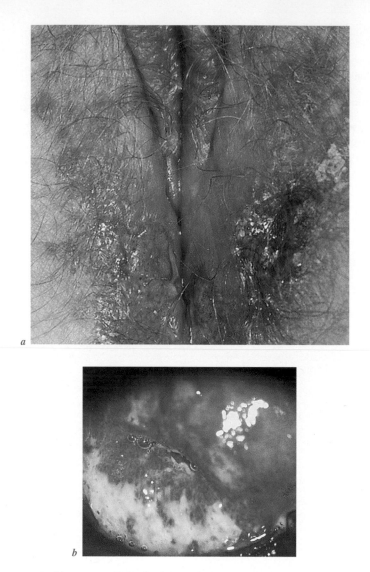

a

b

7–1. *Primary genital herpes.* a. *Multiple, bilateral ulcerative and crusting lesions of the labia and perineum, extending onto the buttocks.* b. *Ulcerative cervicitis. (Part* b *courtesy of Claire E. Stevens.)*

Patient Profile Age 22, single secretary

History Genital and perianal pain, vaginal discharge, fever, and headache for 7 days; boyfriend had recurrent genital herpes, but they carefully avoided sex during symptomatic episodes

Examination Multiple bilateral tender ulcers and crusting lesions, confluent in some areas, of labia majora, perineum, and medial aspects of buttocks; ulcers and purulent exudate of cervix; tender inguinal lymphadenopathy bilaterally; temperature 38.1°C orally

Differential Diagnosis   Genital herpes, syphilis, chancroid

Laboratory   Herpes simplex virus type 2 (HSV-2) isolated from lesions and cervix; syphilis serology, HIV serology, screening cultures for *C. trachomatis* and *N. gonorrhoeae* (all negative)

Diagnosis   Primary genital herpes

Treatment   Valacyclovir 1.0 g PO *tid* for 10 days; patient advised to wear loose-fitting underclothes sprinkled with cornstarch to promote drying and help relieve pain

Comment   Extensive bilateral lesions, inguinal lymphadenopathy, cervicitis, and systemic manifestations indicate primary infection; pain improved after 3 days, completely healed after 2 weeks; counseled about likelihood of both symptomatic recurrences and subclinical shedding, with risk of transmission to future sex partners (but not to her current boyfriend); partner examined and counseled; he was unaware that subclinical viral shedding often occurs between symptomatic recurrent episodes of genital herpes and often accounts for HSV transmission

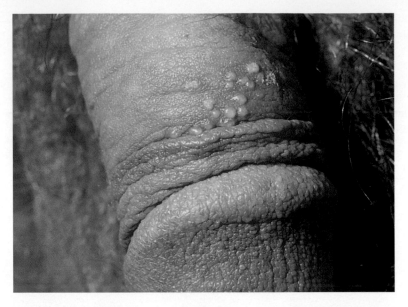

7–2. *Classic vesicular lesions of recurrent genital herpes.*

Patient Profile   Age 38, radiology technician

History   Penile "blisters" for 2 days, preceded by 1 day of itching; two previous similar episodes since initial genital herpes diagnosed 8 months previously

Examination   Cluster of vesicular lesions of penis; no lymphadenopathy

Diagnosis   Recurrent genital herpes

Laboratory   HSV-2 isolated from lesions

Treatment   Valacyclovir 500 mg PO daily as suppressive therapy

Comment   Pain and pruritus resolved over next 3 days; lesions became pustular, then crusted, and healed over 10 days; patient counseled about options of episodic or suppressive antiviral therapy and chose the latter; he remained symptom-free for next 6 months

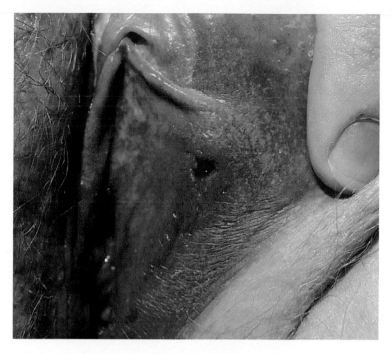

7–3. *Genital herpes: asymptomatic ulcerative lesion of labia minor.*

Patient Profile   Age 28, flight attendant

History   Asymptomatic; sought health care after partner informed her he had gonorrhea

Examination   Nontender ulcer of labia minor, without erythema, purulent exudate, or other in-flammatory signs; otherwise normal

Differential Diagnosis   Herpes, syphilis, chancroid, traumatic lesion

Laboratory   HSV-2 isolated from lesion; darkfield examination negative; type-specific serology positive for antibody to HSV-2; syphilis and HIV serologies negative; *N. gonorrhoeae* and *C. trachomatis* isolated from cervix

Diagnosis   Subclinical recurrent genital herpes; uncomplicated gonorrrhea and chlamydial infection

Treatment   No treatment for genital herpes; cefixime 400 mg orally (single dose) and azithromycin 1.0 g orally (single dose)

Comment   Although patient initially denied symptoms of herpes, after palpating lesion she stated she occasionally felt a painless "bump" in the same spot; positive HSV-2 serology indicated chronic infection; 3 months later patient noted similar lesion and again was culture-positive for HSV-2, and was then prescribed suppressive antiviral therapy; illustrates unrecognized but not truly asymptomatic recurrent herpes

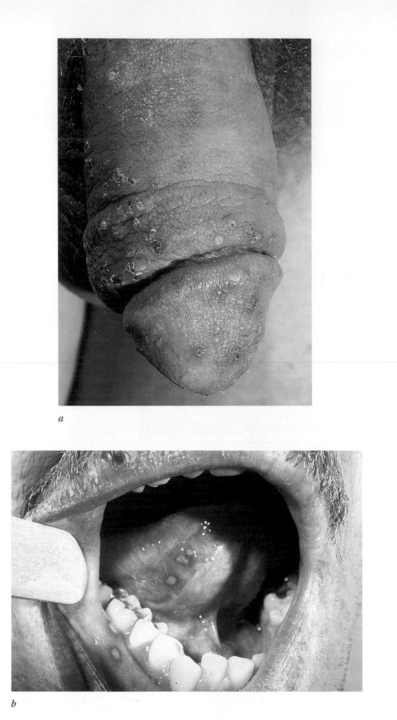

a

b

7–4. *Primary genital and oral herpes:* a. *Pustular and crusting lesions and crusts of penis, with edema of penile shaft.* b. *Oral ulcers. HSV-2 was isolated from both genital and oral lesions. Patient also complained of severe sore throat and fever. When oral HSV-2 infection is seen, it usually accompanies primary genital herpes; oral HSV-2 rarely causes symptomatic recurrences.*

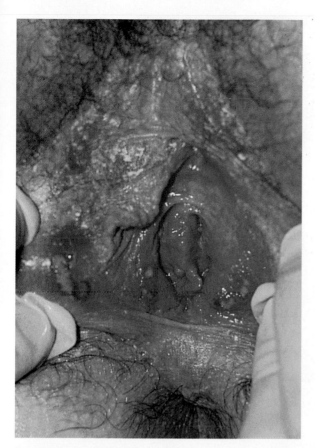

a

7–5. *Primary genital herpes.* a. *Multiple introital ulcers.* b. *Ulcerative cervicitis. (Courtesy of Claire E. Stevens and Lawrence Corey, M.D.)*

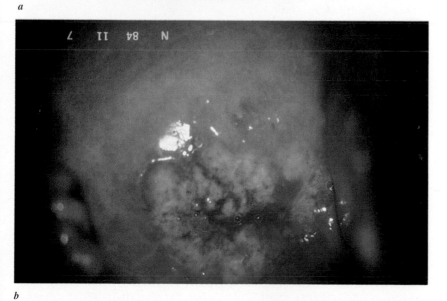

b

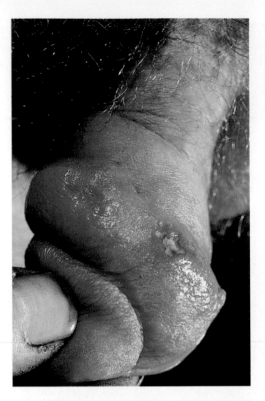

7–6. *Primary genital herpes, showing ulcerative lesions with penile edema. "Penile venereal edema" can accompany herpes as well as urethritis; compare with Figs. 7–4a, 3–8, and 14–3.*

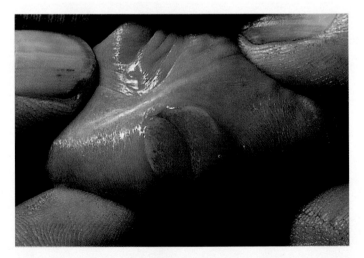

7–7. *Meatal ulceration in a man with urethritis due to primary herpes (same patient as Fig. 7–6). Urethritis is a common manifestation of primary herpes in men and often causes severe dysuria.*

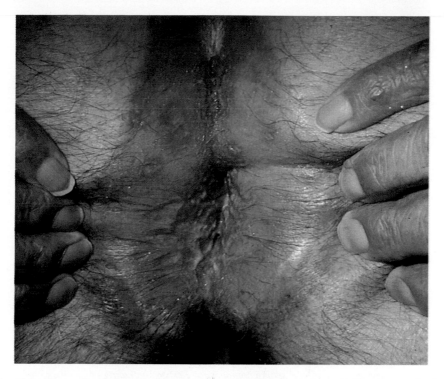

7–8. *Extensive perianal ulcerations due to primary herpes in a gay man. The patient also had fever and tenesmus, and anoscopy showed ulcerative proctitis. HSV-2 was isolated.*

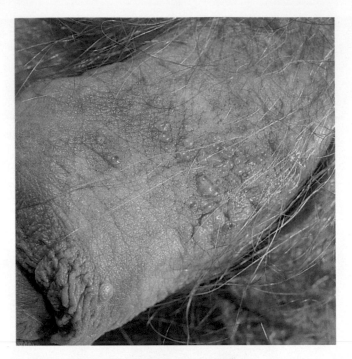

7–9. *Primary genital herpes. The clear fluid-filled vesicles with erythema illustrate the classic sign of "dew drop on a rose petal," pathognomonic for herpes (including chickenpox and shingles). A papular penile wart also is visible.*

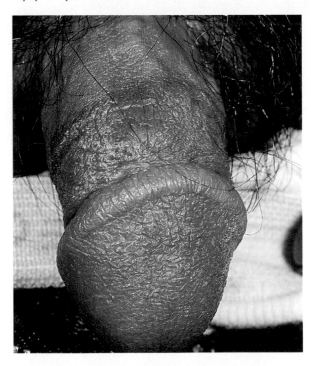

7–10. *"Nonspecific" ulcerative lesions due to subclinical recurrent herpes. The patient was asymptomatic until found to be HSV-2-seropositive and counseled to be on the alert for lesions.*

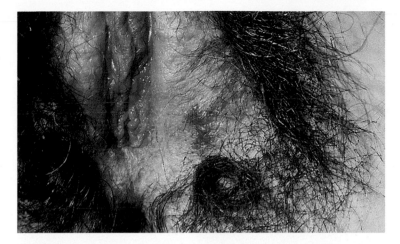

7–11. *"Nonspecific" labial ulcer in recurrent genital herpes. Many recurrent herpes lesions lack the vesiculopustular characteristics of classic herpes.*

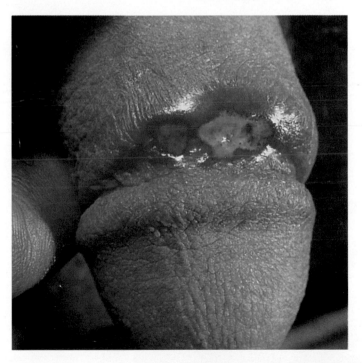

7–12. *Primary genital herpes mimicking chancroid, presenting 1 week after fellatio by a woman with history of oral herpes. HSV-1 was isolated from lesion and culture for* H. ducreyi *was negative.*

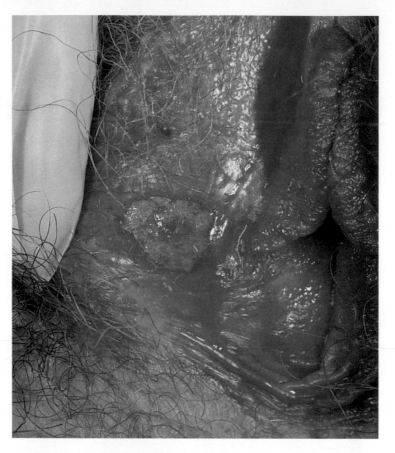

7–13. *Initial, nonprimary genital herpes, with a single introital ulcer. (The violaceous lesion anterior to the ulcer is a hemangioma.)*

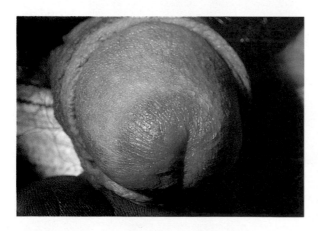

7–14. *Recurrent genital herpes. On close inspection, a small ulcer can be seen in the center of the area of edema and erythema.*

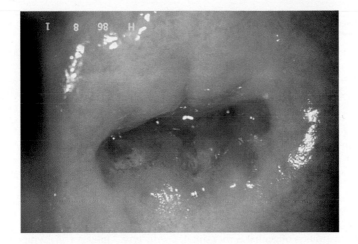

7–15. *Atypical HSV-2 culture-positive ulcers in cervical os in an asymptomatic woman; most subclinical shedding from the cervix is not accompanied by visible ulceration. (Courtesy of Claire E. Stevens.)*

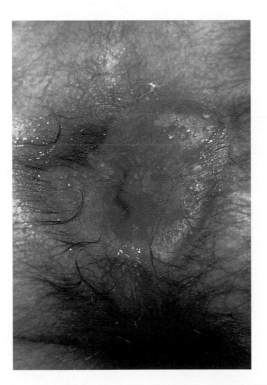

7–16. *Chronic erosive perianal herpetic lesion in a man with AIDS. (Also see Fig. 10–8.)*

ADDITIONAL READING

Brown ZA et al: The acquisition of herpes simplex virus during pregnancy. *N Engl J Med* 337:509–515, 1997. *Prospective study of several thousand pregnant women, showing highest rate of neonatal infection following initial maternal genital herpes.*

Corey LC, Handsfield HH: Genital herpes and public health: addressing a global problem. *JAMA* 283:791–794, 2000. *Summary of public health aspects of genital herpes and recommendations for prevention strategies and research.*

Langenberg AG et al: A prospective study of new infection with herpes simplex virus type 1 and type 2. *N Engl J Med* 342:1432–1438, 1999. *Study of 2,400 sexually active, HSV-2-seronegative persons, showing annual acquisition rates of 1.6% for HSV-1 (mostly symptomatic) and 5.1% for HSV-2 (37% symptomatic); genital and oropharyngeal initial HSV-1 infections were equally frequent.*

Wald A: New therapies and prevention strategies against genital herpes. *Clin Infect Dis* 28 (Suppl 1): S4-S13, 1999. *Review of management strategies for genital herpes developed as background for CDC's 1998 STD Treatment Guidelines*

Wald A, et al: Reactivation of genital herpes simplex virus type 2 infection in asymptomatic seropositive persons. *N Engl J Med* 342:844–850, 2000. *One of several studies by the premier investigators of subclinical genital herpes, showing high rates of subclinical viral shedding in both symptomatic and asymptomatic persons with HSV-2 infection.*

Chapter 8
HUMAN PAPILLOMAVIRUS INFECTION AND GENITAL WARTS

Infection with human papillomavirus (HPV), long considered an inconvenient but benign condition, has emerged as one of the most common and important STDs. Collectively, HPV may cause more sexually transmitted infections than any other pathogen; it is likely that most sexually experienced persons both in the United States and worldwide have been infected. Over 100 HPV types are known. The types that cause genital infection comprise two broad classes on the basis of their association with premalignant neoplasia and cancer. "Low-risk" HPV strains, primarily types 6 and 11, cause exophytic anogenital warts but are infrequently implicated in dysplasia and cancer. "High-risk" types, especially types 16, 18, 31, 45, and several others, cause dysplasia and cancer of the cervix, anus, penis, and vulva; both epidemiologic and laboratory data have firmly established that HPV is the direct cause of these malignancies. For all HPV types, subclinical infections greatly outnumber those that lead to neoplasia or warts.

Often considered to be a lifelong infection, evolving data suggest that both spontaneous resolution and infection with new HPV types are common. Reinfection with the same HPV type, however, appears to be infrequent, probably owing to acquired immunity. Because no treatment has been shown to eliminate the virus from infected skin and mucous membranes, the primary goals for management of genital HPV infections are elimination of symptomatic warts, surveillance for malignancy and premalignant changes, and counseling to limit psychosocial distress. Preventing transmission has been an elusive goal, but active research is underway on HPV vaccines, and immunization may hold promise for prevention, treatment, or both.

EPIDEMIOLOGY

Incidence and Prevalence Estimated incidence 5 million genital HPV infections annually in the United States; >50% of women and probably a similar proportion of men acquire genital HPV during their first few sexual relationships; most infections apparently resolve spontaneously, typically after 6–12 months; total prevalence estimated at >25 million infected persons; HPV DNA can be detected in cervix, vulva, or anus in ≥50% of women attending STD clinics; anal HPV infection is present in >50% of MSM, including 90% of those with HIV infection

Transmission Sexual contact, probably enhanced by friction or microtrauma; perinatal transmission to infants born to infected mothers; autoinoculation from nongenital sites or fomite transmission probably uncommon, but poorly studied

Age Most infections acquired by persons <30 years old, probably reflecting sexual behavior and acquired immunity

Sex No specific predilection known for HPV infection; cervical cancer incidence about 8 per 100,000 U. S. women, fourfold lower than the rate before institution of routine cervical cytology; estimated 5,000 cervical cancer deaths annually in the United States, much higher in developing countries and other settings where Papanicolaou (Pap) smears are not routine

Sexual Orientation Anogenital infection with both high- and low-risk types common in both MSM and WSW; among MSM, annual anal cancer rate estimated at 35 per 100,000 (similar to cervical cancer rate before routine Pap smears); rates probably higher in HIV-infected MSM

Other Risk Factors Immunodeficiency induced by HIV is associated with recrudescence of macroscopic warts and probably accelerated progression of neoplasia

HISTORY

Incubation Period Most infections remain subclinical; exophytic warts typically appear 1–3 months after exposure, but often longer; progression of high-risk HPV infection to cervical, anal, or cutaneous dysplasia or carcinoma in situ typically requires 5–30 years, but rarely <1 year

Symptoms Usually asymptomatic, often detected incidentally by physical examination or Pap smear; visible warts, without pain or discomfort, are most common complaint; large or traumatized warts may ulcerate or become secondarily infected, with itching, pain, discharge, or malodor; urethral warts in men may cause altered urine stream and rarely outflow obstruction; HPV-related vulvar intraepithelial neoplasia (VIN) sometimes pruritic

Epidemiologic History Many persons with subclinical HPV infection lack recent behavioral STD risks; most patients with new anogenital warts have histories of recent sex with new partners.

PHYSICAL EXAMINATION

There are four varieties of exophytic warts:

- *Condylomata acuminata* (singular, *condyloma acuminatum*) usually involve moist or partially keratinized surfaces (e.g., introitus, anus, under foreskin); typical "cauliflower" appearance; hand-held magnification shows central venules in frondlike excrescences
- *Keratotic warts* have horny, often cauliflower-like appearance, typically on dry skin (e.g., penile shaft, scrotum, labia majora)
- *Papular warts* have smooth surfaces, less horny than keratotic warts
- *Flat warts* are macular, sometimes faintly raised, usually invisible to naked eye

Examination usually normal, with infection revealed only by cytology, biopsy, or HPV DNA testing; flat warts sometimes can be visualized by applying 3% acetic acid, resulting in "acetowhite" opacification, but both false-negative and false-positive results common, routine use not recommended; colposcopy useful in women with suspected dysplasia to guide biopsy, but not indicated for routine HPV diagnosis; less common malignant or premalignant HPV lesions include papules (bowenoid papulosis, often similar in appearance to papular warts), white macules or papules of leukoplakia or vulvar intraepithelial neoplasia, and overt genital skin cancer

LABORATORY DIAGNOSIS

Typical changes on Pap stain of cytologic specimens from cervix or anus; on Pap smear, high-grade squamous intraepithelial lesions (HSIL), low-grade lesions (LSIL), or carcinoma in situ almost always indicate HPV infection; HSIL is equivalent to cervical intraepitheliol neoplasia class 2 (CIN 2) or class 3 (CIN 3) and encompasses the abnormalities previously termed *moderate dysplasia,* severe dysplasia, and carcinoma in situ; atypical squamous or glandular cells of undetermined significance (ASCUS, AGUS) may also denote HPV infection; commercially available HPV DNA tests appear highly sensitive and may have important roles in management of women with cervical Pap smears showing ASCUS or AGUS, but not currently recommended for primary HPV diagnosis; periodic Pap smears indicated for all sexually active women; cervical Pap smear currently recommended annually, although less frequent intervals (e.g., every 3 years) may be adequate; studies underway to determine utility of anal Pap smears in screening MSM for anal dysplasia and cancer; current serologic tests have insufficient performance for clinical diagnosis, although useful for epidemiologic research

DIAGNOSIS OF ANOGENITAL WARTS

Visual diagnosis adequate for most exophytic warts; laboratory documentation reliable from experienced laboratorians, but negative results may not exclude infection; biopsy indicated for pigmented and other atypical lesions, those that do not respond to treatment or that have clinical appearance suggestive of malignancy or premalignant changes (e.g., bowenoid papulosis, leukoplakia, giant condylomata); differential diagnosis includes other HPV-related malignant and premalignant conditions, molluscum contagiosum (Chap 9), pearly penile papules (Chap. 21), skin tags, Tyson's glands and other anatomic variants, hemangiomas, condylomata lata of syphilis (Chap. 4).

TREATMENT

Principles Primary goal is ablation of overt warts; no available therapy has been shown to eradicate HPV and none documented to reduce risk of later dysplasia or cancer; many experts believe eliminating visible warts may reduce risk of transmission, but no data available; most wart treatments have 60–80% efficacy with repeated treatment, but highly variable in different patients; recurrences common following all therapies; treatment not indicated for subclinical infection, whether due to high-risk or low-risk HPV types; management of dysplasia depends on degree of dysplasia, regardless of whether or not HPV is documented

Management of Abnormal Cervical Cytology HPV DNA testing may have role in management of some abnormal cervical Pap smears; colposcopy with biopsy indicated for all women with HSIL, CIN 2, or CIN 3, regardless of whether HPV is documented; for ASCUS, recent data suggest colposcopy indicated if positive for high-risk HPV type, because some such women have HSIL on biopsy, but follow-up cytology is sufficient if HPV-negative; such "reflex" HPV testing requires liquid medium Pap smear technology; HPV DNA tests are under study to assess utility as alternative to cytology for dysplasia/cancer screening, especially in resource-poor settings (e.g., developing countries)

Treatment of Anogenital Warts

PROVIDER-APPLIED THERAPY

- Cryotherapy with liquid nitrogen, using commercial directed-spray device, or cryoprobe; repeat weekly as needed; 2–4 treatments usually required; main side effects are local irritation and ulceration
- Podophyllin resin, 10–25% in tincture of benzoin; minimize contact with uninvolved tissue; instruct patient to wash off the resin 1–4 h after application; repeat weekly as needed; several treatments usually required; primary side effects are local irritation and ulceration; contraindicated in pregnancy
- Trichloroacetic acid or bichloroacetic acid, 80–90% solution; carefully avoid contact with uninvolved tissue; repeat weekly as needed; several treatments usually required; local irritation and ulceration are primary side effects
- Alternative regimens, which require special training scissor excision, tangential shave excision, curettage, electosurgery, laser surgery; single treatment usually effective; interferon available but toxic, not recommended; topical 5-fluorouracil no longer recommended because of toxicity

PATIENT-APPLIED TREATMENTS

- Imiquimod 5% cream applied to warts once daily at bedtime; wash off after 6–10 h; repeat 3 times weekly for up to 16 weeks; more effective in women than men, probably because most effective for less keratinized warts and those on moist surfaces; resolution often slower than with other therapies; possibly lower recurrence rate; local irritation common but usually mild; safety in pregnancy unknown
- Podofilox 0.5% solution or gel applied *bid* for 3 consecutive days, followed by 4 treatment-free days, repeated weekly up to 4 cycles; local irritation common; safety in pregnancy unknown

TREATMENT OF MUCOSAL WARTS

- Vaginal warts: Cryotherapy with liquid nitrogen; cryoprobe contraindicated (risk of perforation); trichloroacetic or bichloroacetic acid; podophyllin resin
- Urethral warts: Cryotherapy with liquid nitrogen; podophyllin resin
- Anal and rectal warts: Cryotherapy with liquid nitrogen; trichloroacetic or bichloroacetic acid; surgical excision
- Oral warts: Cryotherapy with liquid nitrogen; surgical excision

Follow-up Routine follow-up not indicated after visible warts resolved

Counseling Advise patients that most HPV infections are subclinical and remain so; that cancer and other complications are rare; that most sexually active persons have been infected, regardless of symptoms or Pap smear results; that infectivity cannot be precisely predicted nor transmission entirely prevented, short of permanent sexual abstinence; that condoms may help prevent some infections, but actual efficacy unknown; condoms not routinely recommended for HPV prevention, even among HPV-discordant couples, except in presence of overt warts; sexual transmission occurs among WSW

PREVENTION

Ablation of overt warts may reduce viral load and perhaps transmission risk, but no data available; sex partners should be examined if they have lesions suggestive of overt warts, but value of routine evaluation of asymptomatic partners is controversial; patients with newly acquired warts should be screened for HIV, *C. trachomatis,* and other locally prevalent STDs; no data support need or efficacy of routine condom use for patients with subclinical infection to prevent HPV transmission; periodic Pap smears indicated for all sexually active women, including WSW, regardless of prior warts or HPV infection

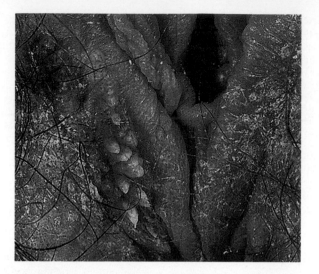

8–1. *Genital warts of labia majora and perineum; lesions have features of both condylomata acuminata and keratotic warts.*

Patient Profile   Age 23, single graduate student

History   Painless genital "bumps" for 1 month; monogamous in a relationship that began 4 months earlier

Examination   "Cauliflower-like" excrescences, some with horny surface, of labia majora and perineum

Diagnosis   Genital warts (condylomata acuminata and keratotic warts)

Laboratory   Routine screening for other STDs, including VDRL and HIV serology, cervical culture for *C. trachomatis*; Pap smear done 4 months earlier, not repeated

Treatment   Lesions frozen with liquid nitrogen spray; repeat treatments scheduled weekly until resolved

Partner Management   Advised to refer partner if he notices genital warts or other lesions

Comment   Patient expressed concern about cancer risk; counseled that different HPV types are warts and cervical and other cancers are caused by different HPV types; advised to continue annual Pap smears; counseled about potential for recurrence of external warts, but advised that most cases resolve spontaneously over several months, and that later recurrences are possible but uncommon

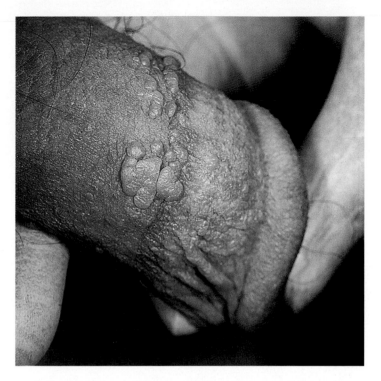

8–2. *Multiple condylomatous and papular warts of the penis.*

Patient Profile　Age 26, single bookstore manager

History　Painless penile growths for 6 weeks; 3 sex partners in past 4 months

Examination　Several 1- to 5-mm excrescences of penile shaft, some appearing "cauliflower-like," others smooth

Differential Diagnosis　Genital warts, molluscum contagiosum, secondary syphilis (condylomata lata), nonpigmented nevi

Laboratory　Screening tests for syphilis, gonorrhea, chlamydial infection, and HIV (all negative)

Diagnosis　Condylomata acuminata and papular warts

Treatment　Cryotherapy with liquid nitrogen, followed by imiquimod 5% cream, self-applied 3 times weekly for up to 16 weeks

Comment　Patient was about to move to another city and requested continued self-applied therapy instead of return for repeat cryotherapy; advised to inform partners to seek examination

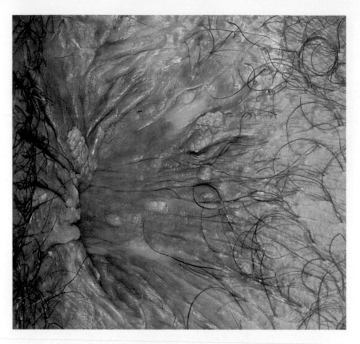

8–3. *Condylomata acuminata of anus.*

Patient Profile   Age 43, gay male television cameraman

History   "Bumps" and anal itching for 1 week; history of anal warts that resolved after treatment with podophyllin 6 years earlier; monogamous for 2 years, denied receptive anal intercourse in past few months; HIV infection diagnosed 2 years earlier, with intermittent medical follow-up (not taking antiretroviral chemotherapy); no fever, weight loss, or other systemic symptoms

Examination   Numerous anal and perianal excrescences with predominantly "cauliflower-like" morphology; anoscopy normal, without visible mucosal warts; general physical examination normal

Differential Diagnosis   Warts; rule out syphilis (condylomata lata)

Laboratory   Stat RPR (negative); rectal cultures for *N. gonorrhoeae* and *C. trachomatis* negative

Diagnosis   Anal condylomata acuminata; HIV infection

Treatment   Cryotherapy with liquid nitrogen, repeated weekly

Comment   Patient advised that reappearance of warts suggests progression of immunodeficiency; urged to resume regular health care for HIV infection; biopsy indicated to exclude anal cancer if incomplete response to therapy

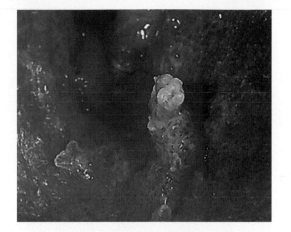

8–4. *Condylomata acuminata of the vaginal introitus, with keratotic changes at the terminus of the largest wart. Central venules can be seen on individual fronds.*

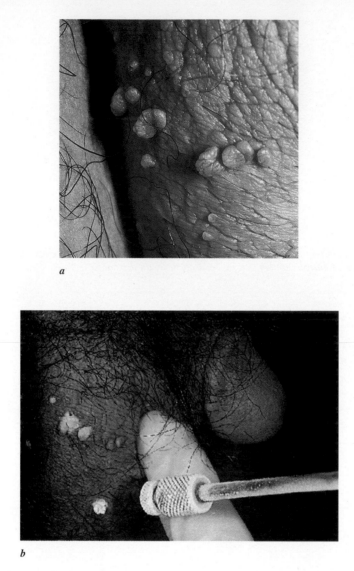

a

b

8–5. *Genital warts of scrotum.* a. *Condylomata acuminata and papular warts.* b. *Cryotherapy with liquid nitrogen.*

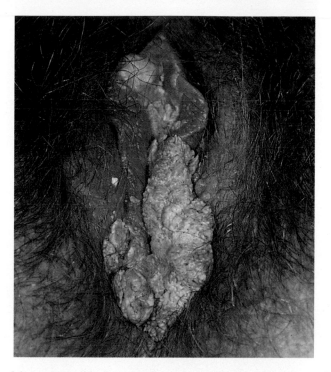

8–6. *Giant condylomata (Buschke-Löwenstein tumor). Malignant changes sometimes occur, and such lesions should be biopsied. Secondary infection and infarction necrosis are common complications.*

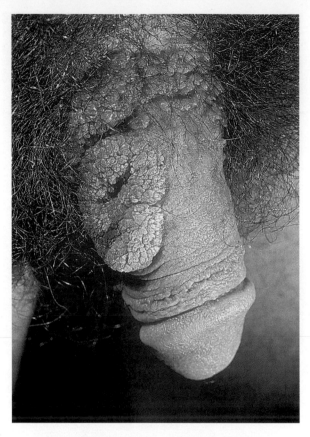

8–7. *Giant condylomata of the penis.*

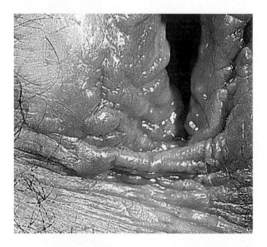

8–8. *Papular warts of the vaginal introitus and perineum.*

3 VIRAL SEXUALLY TRANSMITTED DISEASES

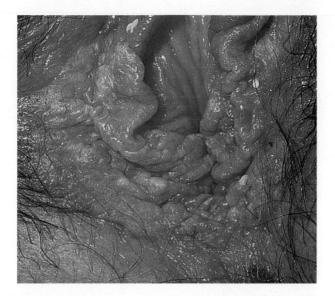

8–9. *Pigmented lesions of vulvar intraepithelial neoplasia with squamous cell carcinoma in situ. (Courtesy of Karl Beutner, M.D.)*

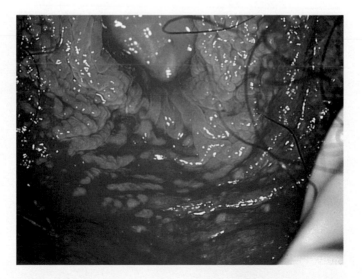

8–10. *Multiple flat and papular warts of vaginal introitus, highlighted with acetic acid solution. Reproduced with permission from KK Holmes et al (eds),* Sexually Transmitted Diseases, *3d ed. New York, McGraw-Hill, 1999.*

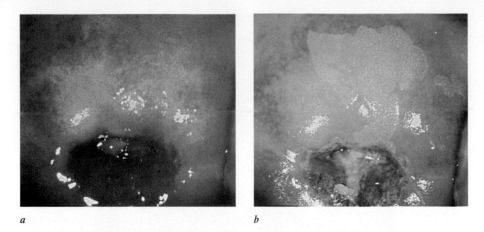

a   b

8–11. *Cervix with subclinical flat wart. a. Normal-appearing ectocervix. b. Flat wart revealed by application of 3% acetic acid, viewed in green light. (Scant mucopurulent exudate also present in os;* C. trachomatis *was isolated.) (Courtesy of Claire E. Stevens.)*

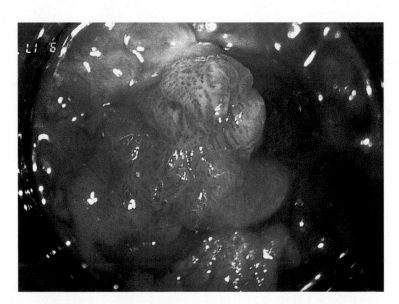

8–12. *Large condylomata acuminata of rectal mucosa, viewed by anoscopy. (Courtesy of Christina M. Surawicz, M.D.)*

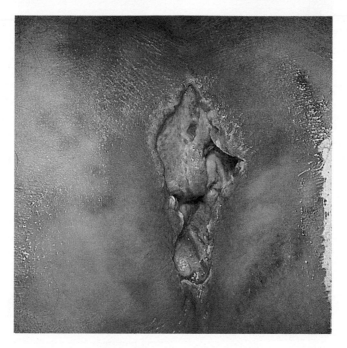

8–13. *Invasive squamous cell cancer of the anus in a man with AIDS. (Courtesy of Steven J. Medwell, M.D.)*

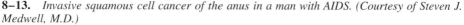

ADDITIONAL READING

Beutner KR et al: External genital warts: report of the American Medical Association Consensus Conference. *Clin Infect Dis* 27:796–806, 1998. *Comprehensive review of clinical manifestations and recommendations for diagnosis, treatment, and prevention of external genital warts.*

Division of STD Prevention: Prevention of genital human papillomavirus infection and sequelae: report of an external consultants' meeting. Centers for Disease Control and Prevention, Atlanta, 1999. *Comprehensive review of HPV epidemiology, relationship to anogenital cancer, and prevention.*

Ho GY et al: Natural history of cervicovaginal papillomavirus infection in young women. *N Engl J Med* 338:423–428, 1998. *Prospective cohort study documenting high rates of both acquisition and spontaneous resolution of HPV infection in sexually active young women.*

Manos MM et al: Identifying women with cervical neoplasia: using human papillomavirus DNA testing for equivocal Papanicolaou results. *JAMA* 281:1605–1610, 1999. *Report of a large prospective study suggesting a role for HPV DNA testing in management of women with Pap smears showing atypical squamous cells of undetermined significance (ASCUS).*

Palefsky JM: Anal squamous intraepithelial lesions: relation to HIV and human papillomavirus infection. *J Acquir Immun Defic Syndr* 21 (Suppl 1):S42–S48, 1999. *Review of anal HPV infection, anal cancer, and interactions with HIV infection in men who have sex with men.*

Walboomers JM et al: Human papillomavirus is a necessary cause of invasive cervical cancer worldwide. *J Pathol* 189:12–19, 1999. *Summary of the etiologic role of HPV in cervical neoplasia.*

Chapter 9
MOLLUSCUM CONTAGIOSUM

Molluscum contagiosum is a common viral eruption that on cursory examination resembles genital warts. Molluscum contagiosum virus (MCV) is related to the pox viruses; two types (MCV-1, MCV-2) have been described. The virus has not been cultivated, perhaps because only relatively mature keratinocytes are susceptible and such cells have not been successfully propagated. In sexually active adults, the infection most commonly involves the pubic area, lower abdomen, upper thighs, or buttocks, as well as external genitals. In young children, the most common presentation is facial lesions, probably acquired primarily through salivary transmission among toddlers. Facial lesions are also common in persons infected or recrudescences of chronic, latent infection as immune surveillance fails. Except in immunodeficient persons, molluscum contagiosum is a benign condition with few complications except for the cosmetic effects, and most cases resolve spontaneously within a few months.

EPIDEMIOLOGY

Incidence and Prevalence No reliable statistics available; accounts for 1–2% of diagnoses in STD clinic patients

Transmission Sexual or salivary transmission; autoinoculation rarely results in local lesions

Age In sexually active adults, most common age 20–40 years

Sex No known predisposition

Sexual Orientation No known predisposition

Other Risk Factors Cellular immunodeficiency

HISTORY

Incubation Period Usually 2–3 months, range 1 week to 6 months

Symptoms Painless papules, often asymptomatic

Epidemiologic History Behavioral risks for STD; sometimes contact with known case

PHYSICAL EXAMINATION

In immunocompetent persons, usually 10 to 20 smooth, waxy papules, often with central umbilication; most common in perigenital areas (especially pubic area), penis, and labia; facial, scalp, and other sites common in children and persons with AIDS.

LABORATORY DIAGNOSIS

No specific tests; characteristic histology if lesion biopsied

DIAGNOSTIC CRITERIA

Usually diagnosed by clinical appearance; may be confused with genital warts on cursory examination; examine small lesions under magnification; expression of hard, white core, usually followed by brisk bleeding, confirms diagnosis.

TREATMENT

Treatment is based on physical ablation of lesions; freezing by liquid nitrogen or cryoprobe is effective; curettage; if few in number, lesions may be unroofed with needle and core manually expressed, although this may carry risk of local reinoculation; podofilox, trichloroacetic acid, and other chemical irritants reported to be effective, but no controlled data available; intralesional interferon may be effective in some HIV-infected patients

SEX PARTNER MANAGEMENT

Some authorities recommend routine referral of sex partners, but others advise patient to refer partner only if symptoms noted

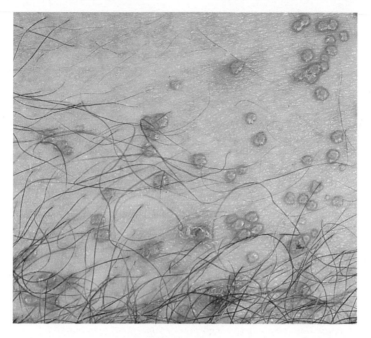

9–1. *Multiple lesions of molluscum contagiosum on lower abdomen.*

Patient Profile   Age 19, male college sophomore

History   Painless "bumps" on lower abdomen and pubic area, first noted 2 weeks earlier; sexually active with new girlfriend for 2 months

Examination   Numerous 1- to 3-mm smooth, erythematous, waxy papules, most with central umbilication

Differential Diagnosis   Molluscum contagiosum, genital warts, syphilis (condylomata lata), other papular eruptions

Laboratory   Screening tests for chlamydial infection, syphilis, and HIV

Diagnosis   Molluscum contagiosum

Treatment   One lesion unroofed and core expressed, to confirm diagnosis; remainder frozen with liquid nitrogen

Partner Management   Advised to refer girlfriend if she notes lesions

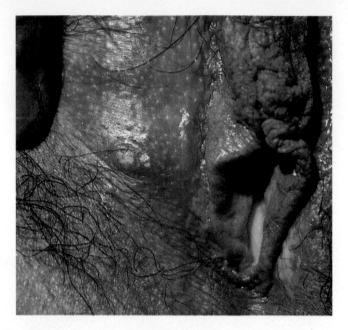

9–2. *Atypical molluscum contagiosum, with loss of superficial epithelium and presenting as a nodular vulvar ulcer. Patient also has discharge due to bacterial vaginosis (see Fig. 18–4).*

Patient Profile Age 20, single, Army-enlisted woman

History Painless vulvar "bump" for 1 week, malodorous vaginal discharge; monogamous for past year, but boyfriend known to have other partners

Examination Nontender, nodular, ulcerated lesion of vulva with firm, white base; homogeneous, white vaginal discharge

Differential Diagnosis Syphilis, genital wart, herpes, chancroid, molluscum contagiosum, granuloma inguinale, cancer

Laboratory Darkfield examination, VDRL, culture for HSV, and screening tests for *N. gonorrhoeae* and *C. trachomatis* (all negative); referred to dermatologist for biopsy; on attempt at punch biopsy, a hard white core was expressed; molluscum contagiosum confirmed histologically; pH 5.0, amine odor test positive, clue cells seen microscopically

Diagnosis Molluscum contagiosum; bacterial vaginosis

Treatment Frozen with liquid nitrogen after core expressed; metronidazole 500 mg PO *tid* for 7 days

Partner Management Advised to refer partner for evaluation

Comment Atypical case; ulcerated molluscum contagiosum rarely recognized

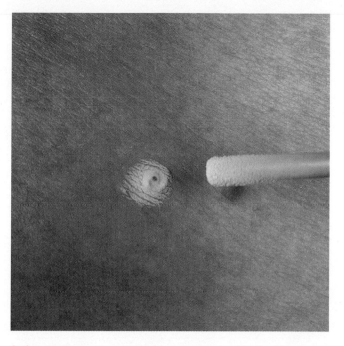

9–3. *Molluscum contagiosum. Freezing with liquid nitrogen spray highlights central umbilication.*

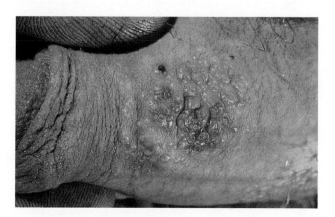

9–4. *Molluscum contagiosum; confluent lesions of penis. Note bleeding after expression of the core of a lesion.*

ADDITIONAL READING

Douglas JM Jr: Molluscum contagiosum, in *Sexually Transmitted Diseases*, 3d ed, KK Holmes et al (eds). New York, McGraw-Hill, 1999, Chap 27. *A well-written, concise review.*

Schwartz JJ, Myskowski PL: Molluscum contagiosum in patients with human immunodeficiency virus infection: a review of twenty-seven patients. *J Am Acad Dermatol* 27:583–588, 1992. *The largest case series of molluscum contagiosum in AIDS patients.*

Chapter 10
HUMAN IMMUNODEFICIENCY VIRUS INFECTION

The acquired immunodeficiency syndrome (AIDS) has become one of the world's major public health problems and by far the most important STDs of all time. The human immunodeficiency viruses (HIVs) types 1 and 2, the causes of AIDS, are transmitted by intimate exposure to blood as well as to sexual and other body secretions, and sex is the most common route of transmission worldwide. HIV-1 is the predominant virus type in the United States. Epidemiologic and laboratory studies have shown that STDs that cause genital ulcers (e.g., syphilis, herpes), many nonulcerative inflammatory STDs (e.g., gonorrhea, trichomoniasis), and perhaps some noninflammatory genitourinary infections (e.g., bacterial vaginosis) enhance the efficiency of HIV transmission and acquisition. It is likely that differences in the background incidence and prevalence of STDs largely explain the marked variations in the frequency of heterosexually transmitted HIV between populations around the globe and across the United States.

All clinicians who provide care to patients with STD or persons at risk should be prepared to recognize the major signs and symptoms of HIV infection and AIDS, elicit histories of high-risk behavior, provide serological testing for HIV infection, educate patients to reduce their risk of exposure, and counsel HIV-infected persons to reduce the likelihood of transmission to others. It is beyond the scope of this book to review all aspects of AIDS or to address the increasingly complex therapeutic aspects of HIV infection and opportunistic diseases. Rather, the focus is on the epidemiology of HIV infection in the United States, prevention, and the recognition and management of early HIV infection.

EPIDEMIOLOGY

Incidence CDC estimates the incidence of new HIV infections in the United States at approximately 40,000 per year; through June 1999, 711,000 cases meeting formal AIDS definition reported; wide variation according to sexual orientation, drug use, and other risk factors

Prevalence As of mid-1999, about 600,000 persons in the United States estimated to be infected with HIV, including 297,000 with overt AIDS; 10–20% of homosexually active men; great geographic variation among injection drug users (IDU), >20% in some cities, <5% in others; 0–5% of heterosexual, non–IDU STD clinic patients

Transmission of HIV Transmitted by sexual exposure, parenteral contact with blood, tissues, organs, breast milk, in utero, or perinatally; worldwide, vaginal or anal intercourse accounts for most infections; occasional transmission by orogenital exposure; transmission by kissing occurs rarely, if ever; sexual transmission and acquisition enhanced by STD, absence of circumcision in males, traumatic sexual practices,

and perhaps bacterial vaginosis (BV), sex during menstruation, and hormonal contraception; male-to-female sexual transmission more efficient than female-to-male; transmission by all routes increased by elevated HIV viral load, (e.g., early HIV infection and advanced immunodeficiency); condoms and other barrier contraceptives reduce risk

Age Reflects peak ages for sexual risks and substance abuse; for overt AIDS, 58% age 25–39 years and 89% <50 years

Sex Most cases occur in men, but both HIV infection and overt AIDS are rising most rapidly in women; for overt AIDS in adults, male:female ratio is 5.1:1 since onset of the epidemic, but 2.2:1 in 1998–1999; 2.7:1 in persons infected by IDU; 1:1.8 among those exposed heterosexually

Sexual Orientation MSM accounted for 48% of cumulative reported AIDS cases in adults through June 1999

Injection Drug Use Sharing injection equipment among heterosexual IDU accounted for 15% of cases through 1999

Heterosexual Exposure   Through 1999, heterosexual exposure accounted for 10% of cumulative adult cases and 40% of cases in women, the most rapidly rising category

Other Risk Factors   Transmission other than by sex or shared injection equipment now rare in industrialized countries; cases attributed to infected blood products, donated organs, or semen now virtually nonexistent in the United States; rare transmission to newborns perinatally and by breastfeeding and to health workers occupationally

HISTORY AND CLINICAL MANIFESTATIONS

Epidemiologic History   High-risk behavior or exposure to known HIV infection; indirect markers include same-sex exposure in men, residence in high-prevalence geographic area, nonparenteral drug use, and past or current STD

Incubation Period   Onset of primary HIV-infection symptoms usually 7–10 days after exposure; without antiretroviral therapy, overt AIDS typically develops 1–10 years (usually 5–8 years) after infection, but sometimes delayed >20 years

Symptoms and Signs

PRIMARY HIV INFECTION   About 50% (range 30–70%) experience mononucleosis-like syndrome, with sore throat, fever, fatigue, malaise, myalgia; sometimes headache, morbilliform rash, lymphadenopathy, mouth ulcers, oral thrush; median duration of symptoms 14 days (range 7 days to 6 weeks)

CHRONIC HIV INFECTION   Following primary infection, most persons asymptomatic until opportunistic diseases supervene; persistent generalized lymphadenopathy without other manifestations does not denote clinical progression; subsequent manifestations highly variable, depending on clinical stage (Table 10–1); manifestations of advancing immunodeficiency and opportunistic diseases include fever, weight loss, diarrhea, seborrheic dermatitis, folliculitis, herpetic ulcers (orofacial, genital, perianal), recurrent anogenital warts, molluscum contagiosum, neuropsychological deterioration, peripheral neuropathy, cough, dyspnea, skin lesions of Kaposi's sarcoma, immune thrombocytopenia, nephrotic syndrome, and many others; common oral manifestations include gingivitis, thrush (candidiasis), hairy leukoplakia of tongue, aphthous ulcers, and lesions of Kaposi's sarcoma

LABORATORY EVALUATION

Tests for HIV Infection

HIV ANTIBODY TESTS   Enzyme immunoassay (EIA) for HIV types 1 and 2, verified by Western blot or other confirmatory test; antibody denotes HIV infection and potential for transmission, except for some newborns in

Table 10-1   CDC CLASSIFICATION SYSTEM FOR HIV INFECTION*

	Clinical Categories		
CDC Categories	**A** **Asymptomatic, Primary HIV, or Persistent Generalized Lymphadenopathy**	**B†** **Symptomatic, without A or C Conditions**	**C#** **AIDS-Indicator Conditions**
(1) ≥500 cells/mm³	A1	B1	C1
(2) 200–499 cells/mm³	A2	B2	C2
(3) <200 cells/mm³	A3	B3	C3

*The shaded portion denotes overt acquired immunodeficiency syndrome (AIDS). By convention, patients do not return to an earlier classification if the condition that resulted in a more advanced classification resolves, with or without treatment.

†Category B clinical conditions include oral candidiasis, hairy leukoplakia, multidermatomal herpes zoster, unexplained fever, diarrhea, or weight loss, and others.

#Category C clinical conditions include *Pneumocystis carinii* pneumonia, Kaposi's sarcoma, ulceration due to HSV lasting >1 month, invasive fungal infections, tuberculosis and other invasive mycobacterial infections, progressive multifocal leukoencephalopathy, HIV-related encephalopathy, HIV wasting syndrome, and numerous other conditions.

Modified from KK Holmes et al (eds). *Sexually Transmitted Diseases,* 3d edition. New York, McGraw-Hill, 1999.

whom passively acquired maternal antibody may be detected for up to 15 months; indeterminate confirmatory tests rare, usually resolved by repeat testing

VIROLOGICAL TESTS Quantitative reverse-transcription PCR assay for HIV RNA currently is the standard test to assess plasma viral load and response to antiretroviral therapy; plasma HIV RNA level predicts transmission risk and rate of progression of immunodeficiency; assays to detect HIV DNA in cells and tissues are research tools but may have occasional clinical application; genotyping or phenotyping of HIV may have a role in predicting efficacy of antiretroviral drugs in individual patients

Assessment of Immunologic Function Primary test is quantitation of lymphocyte subsets; normal CD4 (T4, "helper") lymphocyte count is >600 per mm^3; <200 CD4 cells per mm^3 denotes severe immunodeficiency and is an AIDS-defining criterion (Table 10–1)

Ancillary Tests Tests recommended routinely at initial evaluation of newly diagnosed patients are CBC, platelet count; serological tests for syphilis, hepatitis A, B, and C (HAV, HBV, HCV), and *Toxoplasma;* tuberculin skin test (plus at least 2 controls); chemistry panel, urinalysis, chest radiograph; optional tests, depending on patient's geographic origins and risks, include serological tests for HSV and CMV, plasma *Cryptococcus* antigen, stool examination for ova and parasites

DIAGNOSIS AND CLINICAL CLASSIFICATION

HIV infection is often suspected on clinical grounds and confirmed by serological testing; many cases are diagnosed by serological screening in persons with subclinical infection; as summarized in Table 10–1, asymptomatic persons, those whose only clinical manifestation is persistent generalized lymphadenopathy, and persons with primary HIV infection are categorized as having class A disease; those with specified AIDS-defining clinical manifestations or opportunistic diseases have stage C disease; other symptomatic patients have stage B disease; subgroups 1, 2, and 3 defined by CD4 lymphocyte count; AIDS is defined by stage C or B3 disease

TREATMENT

Antiretroviral Chemotherapy Effective antiretroviral drugs include HIV protease inhibitors (e.g., indinavir, ritonavir, nelfinavir); nucleoside analog reverse transcriptase inhibitors (e.g., zidovudine, didanosine, zalcitabine, stavudine, lamivudine); and non-nucleoside reverse transcriptase inhibitors (e.g., nevirapine, delviridine); combination therapy, usually with a protease inhibitor plus 2 others, lowers plasma HIV RNA level, slows progression of immunodeficiency, apparently prolongs life, prevents perinatal transmission, and probably prevents infection after substantial exposure; many authorities recommend treatment of all infected persons who can tolerate the complex regimens required; others advise waiting until symptoms develop or CD4 lymphocyte count declines to specified levels; drug-resistant HIV probably fostered by intermittent therapy

Prevention of Opportunistic Diseases and Intercurrent Infections If tuberculin-positive without active tuberculosis, give isoniazid 300 mg PO once daily for 1 year; pneumococcal vaccine; annual influenza immunization; antimicrobial prophylaxis against *Pneumocystis carinii* pneumonia if CD4 count <200 per mm^3 and against *Mycobacterium avium* if <100 per mm^3

Post-exposure Prophylaxis Post-exposure prophylaxis with antiretroviral drugs prevents HIV infection following substantial injury with contaminated sharp instruments; efficacy uncertain following sexual exposure; if given, 3 drugs (a protease inhibitor plus 2 reverse transcriptase inhibitors) should be initiated as soon as possible, preferably within 6 hours; probably ineffective if begun >72 hours after exposure; continue treatment for 28 days; repeat serological tests for HIV monthly for 6 months after completing therapy

PREVENTION

Principles Primary measure remains education and counseling to reduce high-risk behaviors, directed to HIV-infected persons, uninfected individuals at risk, and general population; vaccine research underway but effective immunization unlikely to be available in next 5 years; measures to limit nonintimate contact (e.g., quarantine of infected persons, restriction of employment) are unwarranted

Serological Screening HIV testing and counseling widely employed, although efficacy in modifying high-risk behavior remains uncertain; definite benefits include early diagnosis and referral for clinical care; clinicians should routinely recommend serological screening, with pre-and post-test counseling, for all persons with STD or at risk; serological screening of donors prevents transmission by blood products, organs, or artificial insemination; screening of pregnant women has reduced frequency of neonatal HIV infection in industrialized countries

Management of Sex Partners All infected patients should be advised to inform their needle-sharing and sex partners; in some states, clinicians required by law to assure notification of known exposed partners, usually by notifying health department

Reporting Overt AIDS reportable in all states; named reporting of all HIV infections now required in most states.

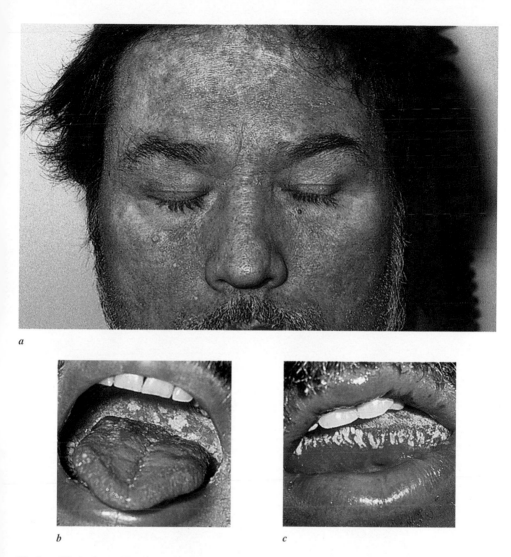

a

b   *c*

10–1. *Clinical manifestations in a patient with AIDS.* a. *Facial seborrheic dermatitis; there is also a lesion of molluscum contagiosum below the right eye.* b. *Oral candidiasis of soft palate.* c. *Hairy leukoplakia of tongue.*

Patient Profile   Age 33, gay male roofer

History   Intermittent fever for 6 months, 15-pound weight loss; skin rash of face for 2 months; sore throat for 2 weeks; occasional unprotected sex with anonymous partners; repeatedly declined HIV testing over preceding decade

Examination   Erythematous facial rash with fine scale, involving forehead, nasolabial areas, and cheeks; umbilicated papular lesion below right eye; patchy white exudate on soft palate; vertically oriented hypertrophic lesions of lateral aspects of tongue

Laboratory   HIV antibody positive by EIA, confirmed by Western blot; VDRL negative; rectal tests for *N. gonorrhoeae* and *C. trachomatis* negative; hematocrit 34%, WBC 4,600 per mm^3 with reduced lymphocytes; CD4 lymphocyte count 122 per mm^3; plasma HIV-1 viral load (quantitative PCR) 88,000 per mm^3; oral swab showed yeasts and pseudohyphae microscopically

Diagnosis   AIDS (CDC stage B3) with oral candidiasis, hairy leukoplakia of tongue, seborrheic dermatitis, and facial molluscum contagiosum

Treatment   Antiretroviral therapy with indinavir, zidovudine, and didanosine; oral fluconazole for thrush; topical ketoconazole for seborrheic dermatitis; molluscum contagiosum lesions treated with liquid nitrogen cryotherapy; trimethoprim/sulfamethoxazole prophylaxis against *Pneumocystis carinii* pneumonia; pneumococcal and influenza immunizations

Comment   After 4 months, patient was asymptomatic, regained lost weight, seborrheic dermatitis and thrush resolved, CD4 count 290 per mm^3; plasma HIV-1 RNA viral load 5,000 per mm^3; *P. carinii* pneumonia prophylaxis discontinued; CDC classification remains B3; by convention, the most advanced classification continues to apply to patients with improved indicators

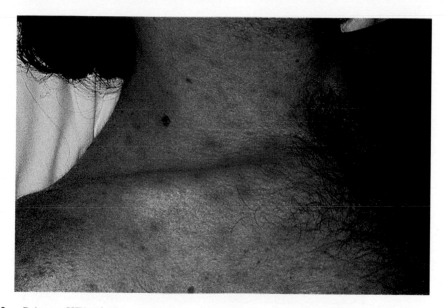

10–2. *Primary HIV infection, with poorly demarcated erythematous macules and papules of the neck and upper trunk. (Courtesy of David H. Spach, M.D. and Philip Kirby, M.D.)*

Patient Profile   Age 24, unemployed gay man

History   Sore throat, fever, and skin rash for 5 days; onset 1 week after unprotected receptive anal sex with unknown partner in a bath house

Examination   Oral temperature 38.3°C; pharyngeal erythema, prominent tonsils with white exudate in tonsil crypts; cervical and axillary lymphadenopathy with 1- to 2-cm, slightly tender nodes; nonblanching maculopapular rash of upper trunk, neck, shoulders

Laboratory   HIV antibody test negative; plasma reverse transcription PCR positive for HIV-1 RNA, 62,000 copies per mm^3; hematocrit 36%, leukocyte count 7,600 per mm^3 with 48% lymphocytes, platelet count 84,000 per mm^3; CD4 lymphocyte count 322 per mm^3; VDRL (negative); rectal cultures for *N. gonorrhoeae* (positive) and *C. trachomatis* (negative); throat culture negative for *Streptococcus pyogenes* and *N. gonorrhoeae*

Diagnosis   Primary HIV infection (CDC stage A2); rectal gonorrhea

Treatment   Patient declined antiretroviral therapy; cefixime 400 mg PO (single dose)

Comment   Typical primary HIV infection syndrome, mimicking infectious mononucleosis; thrombocytopenia often present; HIV antibody test became positive 2 weeks later; fever, rash, and pharyngitis resolved over 2 weeks; over 3 months, lymphadenopathy resolved, differential leukocyte count returned to normal, thrombocytopenia resolved, CD4 lymphocyte count was 665 per mm^3, and plasma HIV-1 viral load 5,500 copies per mm^3; patient continued to decline antiretroviral therapy

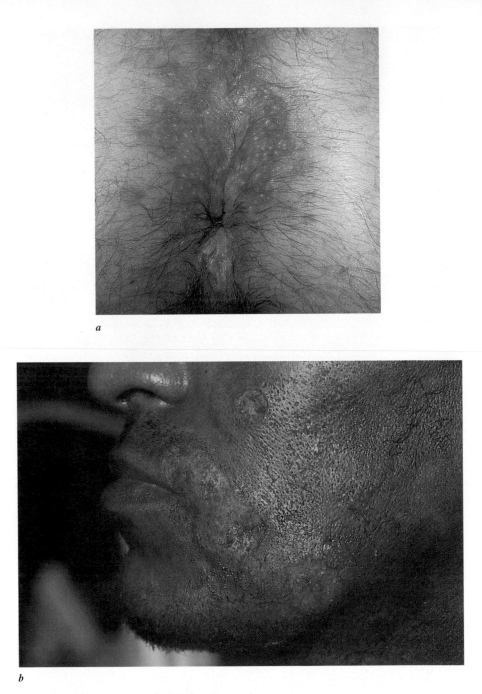

10–3. *Chronic herpes due to HSV-2 in HIV-infected patients. a. Extensive perianal ulceration due to HSV-2; such lesions can be very debilitating due to pain. (Courtesy of Steven J. Medwell, M.D.) b. Chronic facial ulcers due to HSV-1. Lesions usually respond to treatment with valacyclovir, famciclovir, or acyclovir. If present >1 month, such lesions define overt AIDS (CDC class C). (Compare with Fig. 7–16.) (Courtesy of Philip Kirby, M.D.)*

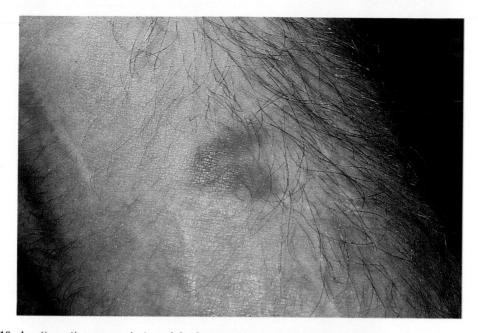

10–4. *Kaposi's sarcoma lesion of the forearm in a patient with AIDS. Kaposi's sarcoma lesions usually are nodular, with violaceous or brown color due to vascular proliferation and hemosiderin deposition, but the appearance is highly variable. Kaposi's sarcoma is caused by the newly discovered, sexually transmitted human herpesvirus type 8 (HHV-8); see Chap. 11. (Courtesy of Philip Kirby, M.D.)*

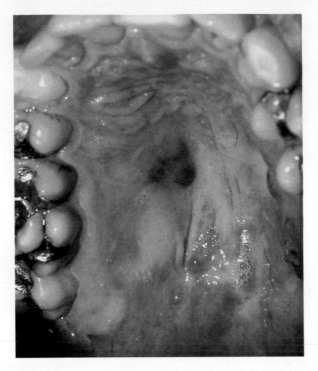

10–5. *Kaposi's sarcoma of the palate in AIDS. Kaposi's sarcoma often presents with oral lesions. (Courtesy of James P. Harnisch, M.D.)*

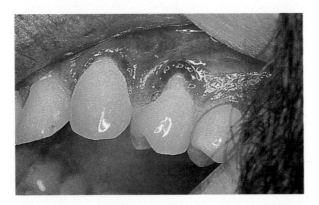

10–6. *Gingivitis in AIDS. Gum retraction and gingivitis are common oral findings in HIV infection.*

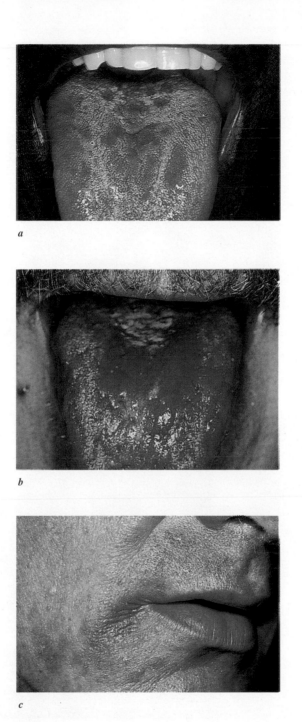

a

b

c

10–7. *Oral candidiasis in AIDS; not all cases present with white patchy exudate typical of thrush (see Fig. 10–1b).* a. *Erythematous candidiasis of tongue.* b. *Erythematous and pseudomembranous candidiasis of tongue.* c. *Angular cheilitis due to Candida albicans. (Courtesy of David H. Spach, M.D.)*

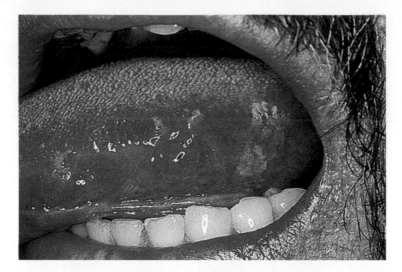

10–8. *Hairy leukoplakia of the tongue in HIV infection; early lesions mimic premalignant leukoplakia and may lack the prominent linear pattern seen in advanced cases (compare with Fig. 10–1c). Hairy leukoplakia is a manifestation of Epstein-Barr virus infection and often responds to therapy with high-dose valacyclovir or famciclovir.*

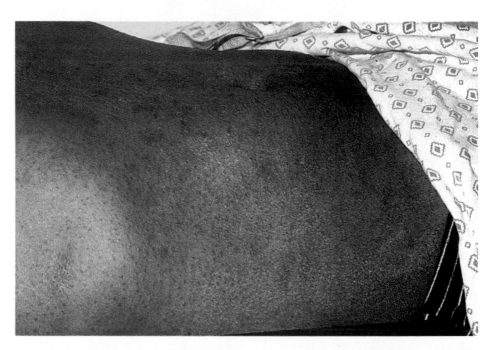

10–9. *AIDS-related ichthyosis. HIV-infected persons with advanced immunodeficiency often complain of dry skin and generalized pruritus. Advanced cases present with overt ichthyosis, with dry, raspy skin, fine scale, and hyperpigmentation. (Courtesy of Philip Kirby, M.D.)*

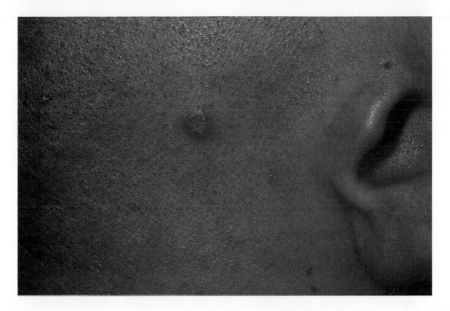

10–10. *Molluscum contagiosum of the cheek in a patient with AIDS. Facial molluscum or warts may result from recrudescence of latent infection, perhaps dating to childhood, due to cellular immunodeficiency. (Courtesy of Philip Kirby, M.D.)*

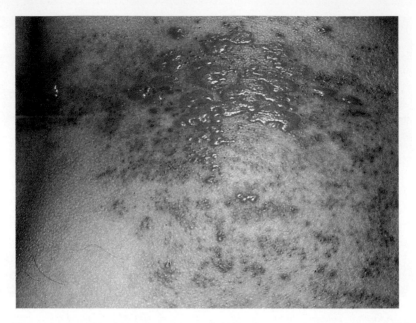

10–11. *Herpes zoster (shingles) in a patient with HIV infection and a CD4 count of 320 cells per mm³. Occurrence of herpes zoster in younger adults raises suspicion of HIV infection. Involvement of more than one cutaneous dermatome is an indicator of CDC class B HIV infection. (Courtesy of David H. Spach, M.D.)*

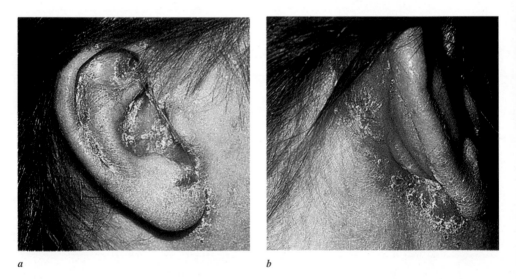

a   *b*

10–12. *Advanced seborrheic dermatitis in a patient with AIDS. Seborrheic dermatitis occasionally is sufficiently severe to suggest herpes zoster. This case resolved promptly with topical ketoconazole therapy. (Courtesy of David H. Spach, M.D.)*

Fleming DT, Wasserheit JN: From epidemiological synergy to public health policy and practice: the contribution of other sexually transmitted diseases to transmission of HIV infection. *Sex Transm Infect* 75:3–17, 1999. *A comprehensive review of the influence of STDs on HIV transmission and implications for HIV prevention.*

Quinn TC et al: Viral load and heterosexual transmission of human immunodeficiency virus type 1. *N Engl J Med* 342:921–929, 2000. *Prospective study documenting the rising risk of sexual transmission of HIV with increasing plasma viral load, and increased risk of HIV acquisition among uncircumcised men.*

Sanford JP et al: *Sanford Guide to HIV/AIDS, 1999.* Vienna, VA, Antimicrobial Therapy, Inc., 1999. *An authoritative, succinct handbook on all clinical aspects of the disease, updated annually.*

Schacker TW et al: Biological and virologic characteristics of primary HIV infection. *Ann Intern Med* 128:613–620, 1998. *The largest series to date of patients with primary HIV infection.*

Spach DH: Clinical management of HIV infection in primary health care, in *Sexually Transmitted Diseases*, 3d ed. KK Holmes et al (eds). New York, McGraw-Hill, 1999, Chap 73. *A succinct review of the clinical manifestations and diagnosis of HIV infection and related conditions.*

Chapter 11
VIRAL HEPATITIS, CYTOMEGALOVIRUS, AND OTHER VIRUSES

Hepatitis B virus (HBV) and cytomegalovirus (CMV), like human immunodeficiency virus (HIV), cause chronic infections and are carried in the blood and genital secretions and are transmitted by blood contact, sexual contact, and maternal–neonatal transmission. CMV apparently is also transmitted through saliva. Hepatitis C virus (HCV) is transmitted primarily by exposure to infected blood; although sexual transmission occurs, its contribution to overall incidence is small and most sex partners of chronically infected persons remain seronegative. All these viruses cause primary infections that are usually subclinical, often followed by chronic infection with the potential for complications years or decades after infection. In contrast, hepatitis A virus (HAV) causes acute hepatitis but rarely chronic infection, if ever. HAV is an enteric virus and is transmitted by sexual practices that foster oral exposure to feces, but not apparently by blood exposure.

HEPATITIS A

Epidemiology and Transmission   Estimated annual U.S. incidence 125,000–200,000 cases; seroprevalence of anti-HAV antibody indicates 15–25% of U.S. residents have been infected; most infections transmitted by fecal–oral contamination, especially among children; sexual transmission is dominant mode among MSM; localized epidemics in MSM sometimes account for most adult HAV cases in a community

Clinical Manifestations   Incubation period usually 3–5 weeks; most adults symptomatic (nausea, malaise, jaundice), but 90% of children asymptomatic; main physical signs are icterus and tender hepatomegaly; clinical resolution occurs and hepatic enzymes usually normal within 6 weeks (rarely up to 3 months) after onset; rare cases of fulminant hepatitis with liver failure

Diagnosis   Based on typical clinical signs and symptoms and hepatic enzyme assays (e.g., alanine aminotransferase, ALT), plus serology for anti-HAV antibody; HAV antigen tests not available; IgM anti-HAV antibody detectable 3 weeks to 4 months after acquisition and indicates acute infection; IgG anti-HAV detectable within 6 weeks of acquisition and persists indefinitely

Treatment   Supportive care; no generally available antiviral therapy known to be effective

Prevention   Anti-HAV vaccine indicated for susceptible (seronegative) MSM, all persons anticipating high-risk exposure (e.g., travel to high-incidence environments), or exposure to known case; usual schedule in adults is 2 doses separated by 6–12 months; within 2 weeks of acute exposure, also administer immune serum globulin IM (0.2 mL/kg body weight); condoms and avoiding practices that foster oral–fecal exposure (e.g., analingus) help prevent sexual transmission

HEPATITIS B

Epidemiology and Transmission   Highly variable incidence and prevalence; estimated 140,000–320,000 new infections annually in the United States; prevalence about 750,000 chronically infected persons; transmitted by blood exposure, sexual contact, and perinatally; sexual transmission probably most efficient by anal intercourse; rates highest in MSM and injection drug users (IDU); about 45% and 15% of all cases in the United States are probably attributable to heterosexual and male homosexual transmission, respectively

Clinical Manifestations   Initial infections often (35–70%) symptomatic, but symptoms usually nonspecific; for overt hepatitis, incubation period usually 6–12 weeks; symptoms and signs of acute hepatitis (nausea, anorexia, jaundice, tender hepatomegaly); 15–20% of patients have serum sickness-like prodrome, with skin rash, polyarthritis, or signs of cryoglobulinemia; chronic infection usually asymptomatic, with or without biochemical or biopsy evidence of chronic active hepatitis, unless cirrhosis or hepatocellular carcinoma supervene

Diagnosis   Usually based on serological tests for HBV surface antigen (HBsAg), antibody to surface antigen (anti-HBs), and antibody to core antigen (anti-HBc); HBsAg indicates acute infection or chronic active infection and potential infectivity; anti-HBs usually indicates resolved or inactive infection; e-antigen (HBeAg) denotes enhanced infectivity and high probability of transmission

Treatment   No curative therapy known; interferon may ameliorate some cases of chronic active hepatitis

Prevention   Immunization is cornerstone; in adults, give three 20-mg doses of HBsAg-based vaccine IM (0, 1, and 6 months); pending universal childhood vaccination, immunize all teens, adults with STD, and health care workers; MSM and IDU should be vaccinated if susceptible; in MSM and IDU, it usually is cost-effective to determine susceptibility serologically, but initial vaccine dose can be given simultaneously with serological test; following acute exposure to known infection, give HBV immune globulin simultaneously with first vaccine dose; condoms probably effective in preventing sexual transmission

HEPATITIS C

Epidemiology and Transmission   Accounts for 15% of symptomatic acute hepatitis in the United States; estimated incidence 30,000–40,000 infections annually; present in 40% of persons with chronic liver disease; mortality 8,000–10,000 persons annually; HCV-related hepatic failure is most common indication for liver transplantation; most cases acquired by blood exposure; sexual transmission probably occurs, but uncommon; no data exist on risks of specific sexual practices or secretions

Clinical Manifestations   Most acute cases are subclinical; chronic persistent infection and hepatitis occur in two thirds of persons with HCV infection, but symptoms and signs usually absent unless cirrhosis or hepatic failure supervene

Diagnosis   Enzyme immunoassay (EIA) for anti-HCV antibody, usually confirmed by recombinant immunoblot assay (RIBA); reverse-transcriptase PCR assay can estimate viral load, sometimes clinically useful; tests to assess hepatic inflammation and function (e.g., ALT, biopsy)

Treatment   Chronic active hepatitis often responds to prolonged (3–6 months) courses of alpha interferon, with or without ribavirin; response depends in part on HCV subtype

Prevention   Cornerstones are anti-HCV screening of blood donors and avoidance of blood exposure (e.g., control of injection drug use, no sharing of injection equipment); condoms and sex partner selection probably have little impact on transmission; routine serological screening recommended for IDU and persons exposed to unscreened blood products; testing not recommended for sex partners of infected persons unless other specific risks exist

CYTOMEGALOVIRUS

Epidemiology and Transmission   Ubiquitous; transmitted by genital secretions, saliva, and blood; vertical (maternal–neonatal) transmission; seroprevalence rises from 10–15% in teens, increasing to about 50% by age 35, but great geographic and demographic variation; superinfection with new strains probably common; nonsexual transmission from infected children to adult caregivers, especially in crowded settings (e.g., daycare, preschool)

Clinical Manifestations Large majority asymptomatic; occasional mononucleosis-like syndrome or granulomatous hepatitis; congenital transmission usually follows primary maternal infection during pregnancy, can cause severe multisystem disease with neurodevelopmental disability, or subtle manifestations (e.g., neurosensory hearing loss); apparent association with atherosclerosis, but causative role uncertain; severe, often life-threatening manifestations (e.g., retinitis, pneumonia, esophagitis, colitis, encephalitis) in persons with AIDS or severe immunodeficiency due to other causes

Diagnosis Culture, antigen, or DNA detection in blood, urine, or genital secretions has limited utility in clinical settings; serology; characteristic pathology on biopsy or cytology, useful for symptomatic disease; except for biopsy for histologic examination, interpretation often difficult because of high prevalence of chronic, asymptomatic infection

Treatment Prolonged therapy with ganciclovir, foscarnet, or cidofovir often effective against retinitis in immunodeficient persons; little documented benefit for other manifestations

Prevention Condoms probably help prevent sexual transmission; no vaccine commercially available; preventing primary infection in pregnant women (e.g., condoms, no new partnerships, avoidance of occupational exposure to young children) probably helps prevent congenital infection; routine screening or partner referral not indicated

OTHER VIRUSES

Human Herpesvirus Type 8 Increasingly known as Kaposi's sarcoma virus (KSV), human herpesvirus type 8 (HHV-8), a newly discovered herpes group virus, is the cause of Kaposi's sarcoma, both in persons with AIDS and in endemic Kaposi's sarcoma typically diagnosed in older persons without HIV infection. Epidemiologic studies and identification of the virus in semen indicate that HHV-8 is sexually transmitted, especially in MSM, although the epidemiology has not been completely characterized and other modes of transmission may be common.

Hepatitis D Virus Formerly known as a "delta agent," hepatitis D virus (HDV) is an "incomplete" virus that causes disease only in the presence of HBV, resulting in clinical exacerbations of hepatitis in persons chronically infected with HBV. HDV is transmitted by blood contact; sexual transmission apparently is infrequent.

Epstein-Barr Virus The cause of classic infectious mononucleosis, Epstein-Barr Virus (EBV) can be transmitted sexually, but most cases are acquired by nonsexual personal contact, probably through exposure to saliva. Recrudescent EBV infection in HIV-infected persons causes oral hairy leukoplakia and rarely more serious complications.

Human T Cell Lymphotrophic Virus, Type 1 Human T cell lymphotrophic virus, type 1 (HTLV-1), causes adult T cell leukemia/lymphoma and tropical spastic paraparesis and myelopathy. HTLV-2 is not clearly associated with known pathology. HTLV-1 and HTLV-2 are epidemiologically similar to HBV and HCV; blood or sexual exposure probably explains most cases.

Enteroviruses Enteroviruses and other enteric viruses are often transmitted by sexual practices that foster oral exposure to feces.

Adenovirus Type 19 Adenovirus type 19 causes acute conjunctivitis with urethritis and sometimes is sexually transmitted.

ADDITIONAL READING

Blauvelt A: The role of human herpesvirus 8 in the pathogenesis of Kaposi's sarcoma. *Adv Dermatol* 14:167–206, 1999. *A comprehensive review of the epidemiology of HHV-8 and its association with Kaposi's sarcoma.*

Centers for Disease Control and Prevention: Recommendations for prevention and control of hepatitis C virus (HCV) infection and HCV-related chronic disease. *MMWR* 47 (RR19):1–39, 1998. *CDC recommendations for HCV prevention, with review of epidemiology and transmission.*

Coonrod D, et al: Association between cytomegalovirus seroconversion and upper genital tract infection among women attending a sexually transmitted diseases clinic: a prospective study. *J Infect Dis* 177:1188–1193, 1998. *A careful analysis documenting 10–12% annual incidence of primary CMV infection in seronegative women attending an STD clinic, and association with acquisition of other STDs.*

Drew WL, Bates MP: Cytomegalovirus, in *Sexually Transmitted Diseases,* 3d ed. KK Holmes et al (eds). New York, McGraw-Hill, 1999, Chap 22. *Comprehensive review of CMV pathology, clinical manifestations, epidemiology, and transmission.*

Lemon SM, Alter MJ: Viral hepatitis, in *Sexually Transmitted Diseases,* 3d ed. KK Holmes (eds). New York, McGraw-Hill, 1999, Chap 26. *Review of HAV, HBV, and HCV from the perspective of sexual transmission.*

CUTANEOUS INFESTATIONS

Chapter 12
PEDICULOSIS PUBIS

Pediculosis pubis, infestation with the crab louse (*Phthirus pubis*), is usually acquired through sexual contact with an infested person, but exceptions are common. The organism grips pubic hair with specially adapted legs and feeds on the patient's blood; intracutaneous bleeding at attachment sites occasionally results in characteristic blue macular lesions called *maculae ceruleae*. Complications are rare, and infestation is more a nuisance than a significant threat to health. Pediculosis pubis is a marker of STD risk, and patients should be screened for other STDs.

EPIDEMIOLOGY

Incidence and Prevalence Very common, but no reliable statistics available; diagnosed in 2–5% of patients attending STD clinics

Transmission Usually requires pubic apposition with an infested person; *P. pubis* is slowly mobile and usually survives < 24 hours without a blood meal; however, exceptions to sexual transmission are common, often explained by exposure to contaminated bedding

Age Reflects sexual behavioral risks

Sex No special predilection

Sexual Orientation No known predilection

Other Risk Factors Communal living, especially in settings with poor hygiene (e.g., shelters for homeless persons)

HISTORY

Incubation Period Ova (nits) hatch in 5–10 days; hatched lice mature in 6–9 days and begin laying nits

Symptoms Visible nits or lice often are the only complaint; sometimes pruritus; lice sometimes are mistaken by patients for scabs in areas of pruritus

Epidemiologic History Behavioral risks for STD; sexual contact with known case; communal living, typically in settings of poor hygiene

PHYSICAL EXAMINATION

Nits, attached at base of hair, are most common and often only sign of infestation; lice may be difficult to find; usually limited to pubic area, but can extend to thighs or trunk; eyelashes occasionally involved, scalp almost never; maculae ceruleae are pathognomonic but uncommon

LABORATORY DIAGNOSIS

If diagnosis is in doubt on visual inspection, characteristic nits and lice may be examined microscopically

DIAGNOSTIC CRITERIA

Identification of nits, lice, or maculae ceruleae

TREATMENT

Permethrin 1% cream rinse, lindane shampoo, or pyrethrins with piperonyl butoxide lotion; applied to pubic area, intergluteal fold, all skin surfaces from knees to waist, and to any other visibly infested areas except eyelashes; reassess after 7 days and re-treat if lice persist or if nits present at hair–skin junction; for eyelash infestation, apply occlusive ophthalmic ointment to eyelid margins *bid* for 10 days

PREVENTION

Main prevention strategies are sex-partner selection and maintenance of personal hygiene; sex partners should be routinely treated

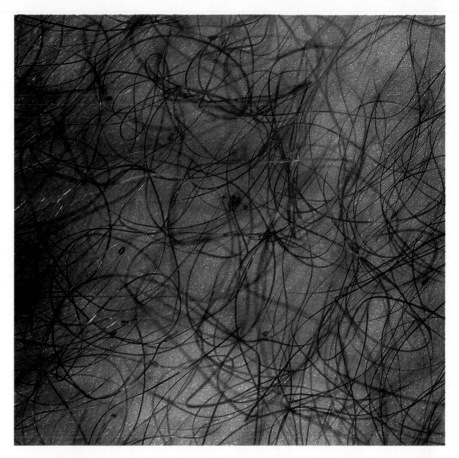

Figure 12–1. *Pubic louse infestation;* Phthirus pubis *and nits attached to pubic hairs.*

Patient Profile   Age 33, male construction worker

History   Pubic area itching for 1 week; noticed "white spots" clinging to pubic hair 1 day earlier; occasional causal sexual contacts

Examination   Nits and typical crab lice in pubic hair; otherwise normal

Laboratory   VDRL, urine LCR test for *C. trachomatis*; patient declined HIV testing

Diagnosis   Pediculosis pubis

Treatment   Permethrin 1% cream rinse

Partner Management   Advised to inform partners and recommend they either attend for clinical evaluation or treat themselves with over-the-counter preparations, e.g., pyrethrins with piperonyl butoxide lotion

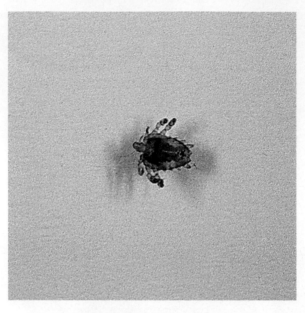

Figure 12–2. Phthirus pubis.

ADDITIONAL READING

Billstein SA: Pubic lice, in *Sexually Transmitted Diseases,* 3d ed. KK Holmes et al (eds). New York, McGraw-Hill, 1999, Chap 46. *A clinically oriented review in the definitive textbook on STDs.*

Chapter 13
SCABIES

Scabies is cutaneous infestation with the itch mite, *Sarcoptes scabiei*. The organism is highly infectious, transmitted by close personal contact; sexual exposure is a frequent but not exclusive mode of transmission. Scabies is among the most common dermatoses observed in persons attending STD clinics. The primary clinical manifestation is an intensely pruritic papular eruption, often with secondary excoriations, but atypical hyperkeratotic, nodular, vesicular, or bullous lesions sometimes occur. These manifestations are mediated by hypersensitivity to the mite and its feces and ova, so that symptoms typically develop 2–4 weeks after acquisition of the first infestation but often within 1–2 days in subsequent infestations. Scabies is sometimes complicated by secondary staphylococcal or streptococcal infection. An uncommon but important complication is crusted ("Norwegian") scabies, characterized by extensive hyperkeratosis and large numbers of mites, sometimes seen in AIDS patients or persons taking large doses of corticosteroids.

EPIDEMIOLOGY

Incidence and Prevalence No accurate incidence data; epidemics tend to recur in 10- to 30-year cycles; diagnosed in up to 5% of STD clinic patients

Transmission Skin-to-skin contact; sexual exposure may be most common mode in young adults, but nonsexual contact in households and other settings (e.g., hospitals, nursing homes, shelters) accounts for many cases

Age All ages affected; most common in young adults and children

Sex Equally common in males and females

Sexual Orientation No special predilection

Other Risk Factors Common in settings of poor hygiene and crowding, such as shelters for homeless persons; nosocomial transmission to health care workers sometimes occurs, especially if initial case has crusted scabies

HISTORY

Incubation Period Typically 2–4 weeks for first episode; often 1–2 days for subsequent infestations

Symptoms Localized or generalized skin rash with intense pruritus, often worse at night or exacerbated by bathing; pruritus sometimes includes apparently uninvolved skin surfaces; absence of pruritus is evidence against scabies

Epidemiologic History Behavioral risks for STD; history of exposure to scabies; communal living, especially in settings of poor hygiene

PHYSICAL EXAMINATION

Papular skin rash, usually with secondary excoriations; often 0.5- to 1.0-cm linear lesions that mark the paths of burrowing mites, sometimes with a leading black dot or small vesicle that marks the mite's location; occasional vesicular, nodular, scaling, bullous lesions or eczematous plaques; secondarily infected pustules or localized cellulitis are common; most commonly involved sites are flexor surfaces of elbows, axillae, hands, finger webs, waist, ankles, dorsal surfaces of feet, genitals, buttocks, inguinal and gluteal folds; penile lesions common, especially of glans in circumcised men; often sparse, with <15 total lesions; crusted (Norwegian) scabies manifested by marked hyperkeratosis, often with fissures and secondary infection

LABORATORY DIAGNOSIS

Microscopy of scrapings of lesions, obtained with a scalpel blade, mixed with 10% KOH solution or mineral oil, showing mites, ova, or fecal pellets (scybala); multiple scrapings often necessary for diagnosis, except in crusted scabies; biopsy occasionally required

DIAGNOSTIC CRITERIA

Diagnosis usually suspected on basis of symptoms and clinical appearance; application of water-based ink followed by alcohol wipe may highlight burrows ("burrow ink test"); microscopic confirmation recommended, especially for atypical cases; assessment of response to treatment (therapeutic trial) sometimes helpful

TREATMENT

Principles Single application of scabicide usually sufficient; therapeutic response may be slow, with persistent pruritus and lesions for 2 weeks or more, due to hypersensitivity to slowly resorbed mites, ova, and scybala; repeated treatment (3 or more episodes) may be required for crusted scabies; ivermectin, a new systemic antiparasitic agent, is effective in 1 or 2 oral doses, perhaps especially useful for crusted scabies and "epidemiologic" treatment of multiple exposed contacts (e.g., in institutions); antihistamines and other antipruritic drugs may speed symptomatic relief; antibiotics sometimes indicated for secondary infection

Antiscabetic Agents

- Permethrin 5% cream, 30 g applied to entire skin surface, washed off after 12 hours; treatment of choice
- Lindane 1% cream or lotion, applied to entire skin surface, washed off after 12 hours; less effective than permethrin, with potential neurotoxic seizures in elderly or children age <2 years old, or in presence of extensive cutaneous disruption
- Ivermectin 200 µg/kg body weight orally, single dose; cure rate may be enhanced by second dose 2 weeks later
- Benzyl benzoate 25% solution, applied topically; usually effective, but not widely used in the United States
- Sulfur in petrolatum applied nightly for 3 days; aesthetically unacceptable to many patients; treatment of choice during pregnancy

Ancillary Measures Launder or dry-clean bed linens and all clothing used within 48 hours prior to treatment; antipruritic drugs or antibiotics, if indicated

PREVENTION

Mainstays of prevention are avoidance of high-risk sexual exposures, shared living quarters in settings of poor hygiene, and direct personal contact with infested persons; routinely treat sex partners and persons sharing living quarters with infested persons

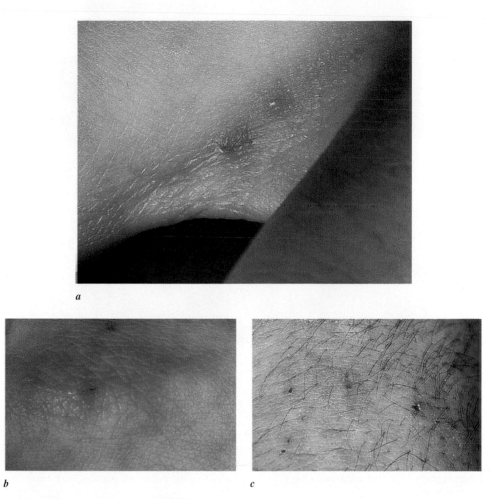

a

b   *c*

13–1. *Scabies. a. Papules (one excoriated) of finger web. b. Papules of knuckle; note dark line across papule, which yielded diagnostic scrapings. c. Excoriations on extensor surface of elbow.*

Patient Profile   Age 19, male carpenter

History   Intense itching "all over" for 2 weeks, worse at night; onset 4 weeks after intercourse with an unknown female partner

Examination   Erythematous papules and excoriations of hands, elbows, around waist

Differential Diagnosis   Scabies, eczema, dermatitis herpetiformis, contact dermatitis

Laboratory   Microscopic examination of lesion scrapings demonstrated ova and feces of *S. scabiei; C. trachomatis* identified by urine LCR test; VDRL and HIV serology negative

Diagnosis   Scabies

Treatment   Permethrin 5% cream; counseled to launder bed linens and clothing used in preceding 48 hours; azithromycin 1.0 g given after *C. trachomatis* identified

Comment   Symptoms and rash resolved gradually over 10 days; incidental chlamydial infection illustrates importance of scabies as STD risk; patient's sex partner could not be located

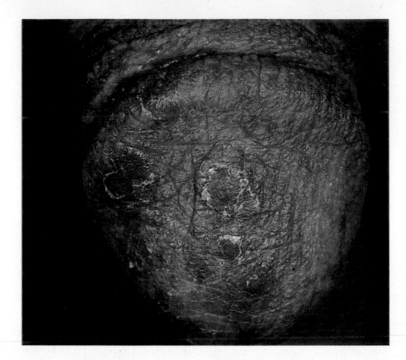

13–2. *Scabies of glans penis. Note similarity to secondary syphilis (Fig. 4–13) and psoriasis (Figs. 21–3 and 21–4).*

Patient Profile   Age 37, homeless man living in a communal shelter

History   Pruritic rash for 2 weeks; worse at night; no recent sexual exposure; scabies or itching reported to be common among other shelter residents

Examination   Exfoliating papules on glans and shaft of penis; numerous papules, nodules, excoriations of trunk

Differential Diagnosis   Scabies, secondary syphilis, keratoderma blennorrhagica (Reiter's syndrome), psoriasis

Laboratory   Scrapings negative for scabies; VDRL, HIV serology, urine LCR tests for *N. gonorrhoeae* and *C. trachomatis* (all negative)

Diagnosis   Scabies

Treatment   Permethrin 5% cream

Comment   Despite negative scrapings, diagnosis based on clinical presentation and epidemiologic history; patient's symptoms and rash resolved over 2 weeks (therapeutic response helped confirm diagnosis); local health department inspected shelter, diagnosed 5 additional cases, and arranged for treatment of all residents and simultaneous laundry of all clothing and bed linens

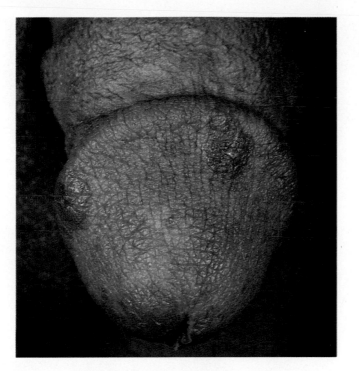

13–3. *Scabies: papulonodular lesions of penis.*

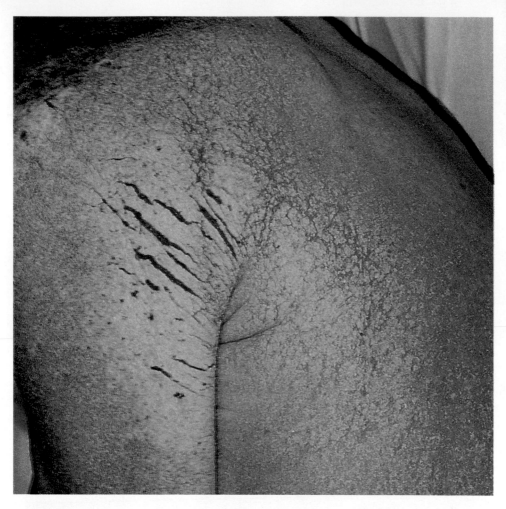

13–4. *Crusted (Norwegian) scabies in a man with AIDS. (Reprinted with permission from Spach DH, Fritsche TR: Norwegian scabies in a patient with AIDS. N Engl J Med 331:777, 1994.)*

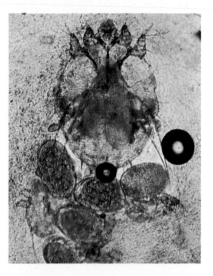

13–5. Sarcoptes scabiei *with ova, scraped from a scabies skin lesion. Reproduced with permission from KK Holmes et al (eds).* Sexually Transmitted Diseases, *3d ed. New York, McGraw-Hill, 1999.*

ADDITIONAL READING

Bigby M: A systematic review of the treatment of scabies. *Arch Dermatol* 136:387–389, 2000. *Review of current therapy, including use of oral ivermectin.*

Platts-Mills TA, Rein MF: Scabies, in *Sexually Transmitted Diseases,* 3d ed. KK Holmes et al (eds). New York, McGraw-Hill, 1999, Chap 47. *A general review in the main STD textbook.*

Routh HB et al: Ectoparasites as sexually transmitted diseases. *Semin Dermatol* 13:243–247, 1994. *Review of scabies and pediculosis pubis, with emphasis on their epidemiologic association with STD.*

CLINICAL SYNDROMES

Chapter 14
NONGONOCOCCAL URETHRITIS

Nongonococcal urethritis (NGU), by definition, is urethritis not due to *Neisseria gonorrhoeae.* NGU is the most common clinical disorder among men presenting to most STD clinics. The term "non-specific" urethritis is discouraged because it fosters the notion that the cause is unknown or un-knowable. Although earlier studies indicated 30–50% of cases were due to *Chlamydia trachomatis,* in most settings chlamydial infection now accounts for 20–30% of cases. The causes of the remaining cases are uncertain. *Ureaplasma urealyticum* may cause up to 20–40%, but conflicting data exist, and neither *C. trachomatis* nor *U. urealyticum* can be isolated from at least one third of men with NGU. Recent research suggests that *Mycoplasma genitalium,* a fastidious, difficult-to-isolate organism, may cause some cases. The association of NGU with oral sex in MSM suggests that oropharyngeal flora sometimes causes urethritis. Fewer than 5% of cases are due to *Trichomonas vaginalis* or herpes simplex virus (HSV); the latter usually is accompanied by external genital herpetic lesions and prominent dysuria. Coliform bacteria occasionally cause urethritis following insertive anal intercourse, particularly in MSM. The differential diagnosis also includes urethral foreign bodies and periurethral fistulas, but both are rare.

Persistent or recurrent NGU is a common problem, often vexing for patients and providers alike. This syndrome apparently is distinct from acute NGU; repeated relapses are common, often without sexual reexposure, and *C. trachomatis* or other recognized pathogens are almost never identified. Although recurrent NGU occasionally may be associated with nonbacterial prostatitis or chronic pelvic pain syndrome, the prostate usually is not involved. Despite historical beliefs, there is no evidence that alcohol, highly spiced foods, physical "strain," or changes in sexual frequency can cause acute or recurrent urethritis or prostatitis. Noninfectious immunologic factors may cause some cases; for example, urethritis sometimes accompanies nonsexually acquired Reiter's syndrome triggered by enteric infection.

The main complications of NGU are those caused or triggered by *C. trachomatis,* including acute epididymitis and Reiter's syndrome, but neither of these syndromes has been linked to nonchlamydial NGU. There is no evidence that urethral stricture results from NGU; most such cases in the pre-antibiotic era probably were due to gonorrhea or to traumatic therapies. Therefore, the most important consequences of NGU are those due to *C. trachomatis* in women. In the absence of chlamydial infection, neither acute nor recurrent NGU has been associated with morbidity in patients' male or female sex partners. Although the partners usually are treated with antibiotics, the need to do so is uncertain if chlamydial infection has been excluded.

EPIDEMIOLOGY

Incidence and Prevalence   Accurate data unavailable; the most common STD syndrome in men, present in 20–30% of men in some STD clinics

Transmission   Initial episodes of NGU almost always acquired sexually; orogenital exposure probably accounts for some cases of non-chlamydial NGU; recurrent nonchlamydial NGU probably results primarily from relapse, not reinfection

Age   Most cases age 15–35; all ages susceptible

Sex   By definition, NGU occurs only in men; mucopurulent cervicitis (see Chap. 17) may be the female counterpart

Sexual Orientation   Occurs in both heterosexual men and MSM; in MSM, *C. trachomatis* accounts for <10% of cases, and many cases associated with orogenital exposure

HISTORY

Incubation Period   Typically 1–3 weeks, sometimes longer; subclinical infection common

Symptoms   Primarily urethral discharge; often urethral pruritus; dysuria usually mild, often absent; severe dysuria suggests herpetic urethritis

Epidemiologic History Usually new sex partner or other exposure history

PHYSICAL EXAMINATION

Urethral discharge, typically mucoid or mucopurulent, but occasionally purulent; many patients lack demonstrable discharge, depending partly on time since urination; occasional meatal erythema; localized tenderness along penile shaft suggests herpes; "penile venereal edema," a rare complication of urethritis or genital herpes, is painless edema of penis, usually without erythema or other inflammatory signs

LABORATORY

Gram-Stained Smear Smear of exudate showing ≥5 PMNs per oil immersion (1000×) microscopic field, in an area of smear that contains maximum concentration of cells in monolayer; absence of gram-negative diplococci

Microbiologic Tests Test for *C. trachomatis,* preferably by DNA amplification test or culture (see Chap. 2); culture or other approved test for *N. gonorrhoeae;* urethral swab, passed 2–4 cm beyond meatus, is preferred specimen for Gram stain and chlamydia and gonorrhea testing; first 30 mL of voided urine acceptable for DNA amplification tests but not culture or other tests; tests for *U. urealyticum* not indicated; patients who have participated in insertive anal intercourse should have urine culture for uropathogens; test for HSV or *T. vaginalis* sometimes indicated by clinical presentation or exposure history

Other Tests Leukocyte esterase dipstick test or microscopy of first 30 mL of voided urine can substitute for Gram-stained smear as evidence of urethral inflammation

DIAGNOSTIC CRITERIA

Diagnosis requires documentation of urethral inflammation, plus either symptoms or signs, or repeated documentation of urethral inflammation; when practical, examine when patient has not voided for ≥4 hours

Documentation of Urethritis

- Urethral leukocytosis, documented by Gram-stained smear of external urethral exudate or endourethral swab, showing ≥5 PMNs per 1000× field; or positive leukocyte esterase test on initial 30 mL of voided urine
- Plus *either* (1) a history of urethral discharge, dysuria, or urethral pruritus *or* (2) abnormal urethral exudate on physical examination
- If patient only has urethral leukocytosis without symptoms or abnormal discharge, reevaluate after 5–7 days when patient has not voided for ≥4 hours; repeated evidence of urethral leukocytosis confirms urethritis, despite absence of symptoms and signs

Persistent Urethritis Trichomoniasis sometimes explains urethritis that persists (i.e., no symptomatic improvement) several days after start of treatment; confirm urethral leukocytosis; if leukocytosis documented by Gram stain or leukocyte esterase, consider test for *T. vaginalis;* if severe dysuria or other signs of genital herpes, test for HSV

Recurrent NGU After symptomatic resolution, urethritis recurs within 6 weeks in 10–20% of men following chlamydial NGU and in 20–40% after nonchlamydial NGU; confirm urethral inflammation by Gram-stained smear or leukocyte esterase test; repeated cultures for *C. trachomatis,* genital mycoplasmas, or uropathogens rarely are positive and usually are not indicated; repeated courses of antimicrobial therapy not indicated in absence of urethral leukocytosis

TREATMENT

Initial, Nonrecurrent NGU*

TREATMENTS OF CHOICE

- Azithromycin 1.0 g PO, single dose
- Doxycycline 100 mg PO *bid* for 7 days

ALTERNATIVE REGIMENS

- Erythromycin base 500 mg PO *qid* (or equivalent alternate erythromycin formulation) for 7 days
- Ofloxacin 300 mg PO *bid* for 7 days
- Tetracycline HCl 500 mg PO *qid* for 7 days

Persistent NGU Consider metronidazole 2.0 g PO, single dose, for presumptive trichomoniasis; or consider antiviral therapy if HSV infection suspected

*No previous NGU, or ≥3 months since prior episode

Recurrent NGU For first recurrence (in absence of reexposure), treat with doxycycline 100 mg PO *bid* for 7 days if azithromycin or erythromycin was used for initial treatment; give erythromycin 500 mg PO *qid* for 7 days if doxycycline or tetracycline was used initially; for subsequent recurrences, many experts recommend ofloxacin 300 mg PO *bid* or ciprofloxacin 500 mg PO *bid,* for 2–3 weeks; persistent or recurrent symptoms should not be treated with antimicrobial drugs unless urethral leukocytosis is documented

PREVENTION

As for chlamydial infection (Chap. 2); examine and treat female sex partners of patients with nonrecurrent NGU for presumptive chlamydial infection; most authorities recommend treatment of partners of men with initial nonchlamydial NGU; repeated treatment not recommended for partners of men with recurrent NGU; recommend condoms for new or casual sexual encounters

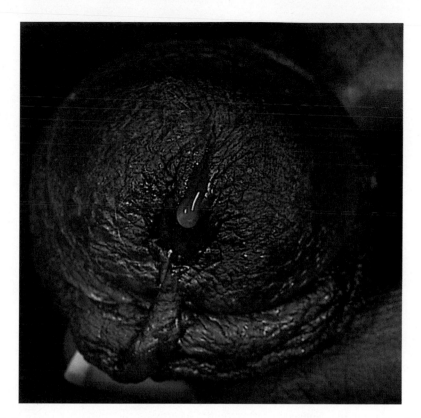

14–1. *Mucopurulent urethral discharge in nongonococcal urethritis. Also see Fig. 2–1.*

Patient Profile   Age 26, heterosexual computer programmer

History   Urethral "itching" and intermittent urethral discharge for 7 days; began a new sexual relationship 6 weeks earlier

Examination   Mucopurulent urethral discharge

Differential Diagnosis   Nongonococcal urethritis, gonorrhea; small likelihood of trichomonal or herpetic urethritis

Laboratory   Urethral Gram stain showed 15–20 PMNs per 1000× field and scant mixed bacterial flora, without gram-negative diplococci; urethral cultures for *C. trachomatis* and *N. gonorrhoeae* (both negative); VDRL and HIV serology negative

Diagnosis   Nonchlamydial, nongonococcal urethritis

Treatment   Azithromycin 1.0 g PO, single dose

Other   Patient counseled about sexually acquired nature of his infection and need to arrange for examination and treatment of partner; follow-up optional if symptoms resolve and partner treated

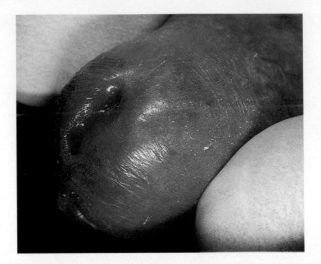

14–2. *Nongonococcal urethritis with scant, clear, mucoid urethral discharge.*

Patient Profile   Age 34, gay flight attendant

History   Urethral discharge for 5 days; no dysuria or other symptoms; periodically has had unprotected oral sex and insertive anal sex with multiple unknown partners in a bath house; denied receptive anal intercourse in preceding year

Examination   Scant, clear, mucoid urethral discharge

Differential Diagnosis   Nongonococcal urethritis, gonorrhea, coliform urethritis

Laboratory   Urethral Gram stain showed 10–12 PMNs per 1000× field, without gram-negative diplococci; urethral and pharyngeal cultures for *N. gonorrhoeae* (both negative); first 30 mL of voided urine tested for *C. trachomatis* by LCR (negative) and cultured for coliform bacteria (negative); VDRL and HIV serology (negative)

Diagnosis   Nonchlamydial, nongonococcal urethritis

Treatment   Doxycycline 100 mg PO *bid* for 7 days

Other   Doxycycline may be preferred for treatment of NGU in MSM, because experience limited with azithromycin; no effort made to notify partners, because partners unknown and no known benefit to treatment of same-sex partners of men with NGU; acquisition by oral sex may be common in MSM

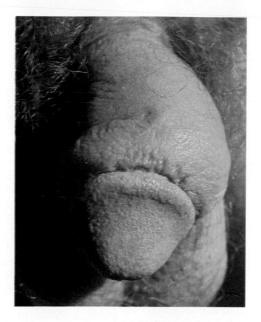

14–3. *Penile venereal edema in a patient with chlamydial NGU. Compare with Figs. 3–8, 7–4, and 7–6.*

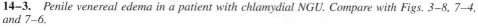

ADDITIONAL READING

Burstein GR, Zenilman JM: Nongonococcal urethritis: a new paradigm. *Clin Infect Dis* 28 (Suppl 1): S66–S73, 1999. *Review of etiology, epidemiology, and treatment of NGU.*

Hooton TM et al: Erythromycin for persistent or recurrent nongonococcal urethritis: a randomized, placebo-controlled trial. *Ann Intern Med* 113:21–26, 1990. *The best treatment study of recurrent NGU, including review of etiology and clinical evaluation.*

Lafferty WE et al: Sexually transmitted diseases in men who have sex with men: acquisition of gonorrhea and nongonococcal urethritis by fellatio and implications for STD/HIV prevention. *Sex Transm Dis* 24:272–278, 1997. *A study showing oral sex to be an independent risk factor for nonchlamydial NGU.*

Schwartz MA, Hooton TM: Etiology of nongonococcal nonchlamydial urethritis. *Dermatol Clin* 16:727–733, 1998. *Review of current research into the etiology of nonchlamydial NGU.*

Stamm WE et al: Azithromycin for empirical treatment of the nongonococcal urethritis syndrome in men: a randomized double-blind study *JAMA* 274:545–549, 1995. *A randomized, controlled trial showing doxycycline and azithromycin to have similar efficacies for treatment of both chlamydial and nonchlamydial NGU.*

Chapter 15
EPIDIDYMITIS

Acute epididymitis results from ascending lower urinary tract infection, analogous to the pathogenesis of pelvic inflammatory disease in women. *Chlamydia trachomatis* causes most cases formerly classified as "nonspecific" epididymitis, and many others are caused by *Neisseria gonorrhoeae*. Coliform bacteria or other traditional uropathogens are common causes in older men, men who have sex with men (MSM), and in men of any age following urinary tract surgery or instrumentation. Tuberculosis and systemic fungal infections are occasionally implicated in all age groups. Epididymitis, usually bilateral, is an occasional side effect of the antiarrhythmic drug amiodarone.

EPIDEMIOLOGY

Incidence and Prevalence No accurate statistics available; in heterosexual men <35 years old, 60–80% due to *C. trachomatis* and 5–25% to *N. gonorrhoeae*, depending on local incidences of chlamydial infection and gonorrhea; coliforms account for many cases in MSM

Transmission As for *C. trachomatis* and *N. gonorrhoeae*; coliform infection in men often sexually acquired by anal intercourse

Age Most sexually acquired cases age 15–35 years

Sexual Orientation Increased risk of coliform infection for MSM

Other Risk Factors Urinary tract instrumentation; anatomic abnormalities that predispose to urinary tract infection in men; bacterial prostatitis; amiodarone therapy; physical "strain" (valsalva maneuver that may cause reflux of urine into epididymis) does not directly cause epididymitis, but may sometimes contribute to pathogenesis in presence of predisposing infection

HISTORY

Incubation Period Not well studied; usually follows acquisition of urethral chlamydial, gonococcal, or coliform infection by several days to a few weeks

Symptoms Testicular pain and swelling, ranging in severity from mild to severe; sometimes inguinal pain; symptoms usually develop over 1–2 days, but sometimes suddenly; fever uncommon; symptoms of urethritis reflect underlying etiology (mild or absent in chlamydial infection, usually prominent in gonorrhea); urgency or urinary frequency without discharge suggest coliform as causative agent

Epidemiologic History Often high-risk sexual exposure (e.g., new partner, symptomatic partner, insertive anal sex)

PHYSICAL EXAMINATION

Epididymal and testicular enlargement; tenderness, often severe, typically localized to epididymis but may involve testicle as well as epididymis (epididymo-orchitis); usually unilateral; sometimes scrotal erythema; signs of urethritis often present

LABORATORY TESTS

Evaluation for Lower Genital Tract Infection As for NGU or gonorrhea (see Chaps. 2, 3, and 14); midstream urine may show pyuria by microscopy or leukocyte esterase test

Microbiologic Tests Urethral specimen for *C. trachomatis* and *N. gonorrhoeae* culture, DNA amplification assay, or other sensitive test (see Chaps. 2 and 3); midstream urine culture for uropathogens

Other Tests Stat assessment of blood flow (e.g., Doppler or technetium 99m scan) in patients at risk for testicular torsion, including all adolescents, patients with sudden onset, absence of urethritis or pyuria, or if testicle elevated in scrotal sac; blood cultures if febrile

DIAGNOSIS

Epididymal or testicular tenderness and swelling plus evidence of urethritis or bacterial urinary tract infection; differential diagnosis includes the "four Ts": *T*orsion (common in teens, many of whom also are at risk for STD), *T*umor (i.e., testicular cancer, a common malignancy in young men), *T*rauma (usually with history of specific injury), and *T*uberculosis; other uncommon causes of epididymitis include cryptococcosis and other systemic fungal infections and amiodarone toxicity; inguinal hernia occasionally can be confused with epididymitis

TREATMENT

Presumptive Therapy for Sexually Acquired Epididymitis

- Ofloxacin 300 mg PO *bid* for 10 days (or other fluoroquinolone active against *C. trachomatis*)

- Ceftriaxone 250 mg IM plus doxycycline, 100 mg *bid* for 10 days

- Ofloxacin or other fluoroquinolone also indicated when clinical and epidemiologic data suggest coliform epididymitis; for causes other than *N. gonorrhoeae* or *C. trachomatis,* adjust therapy as needed on basis of antimicrobial susceptibility tests

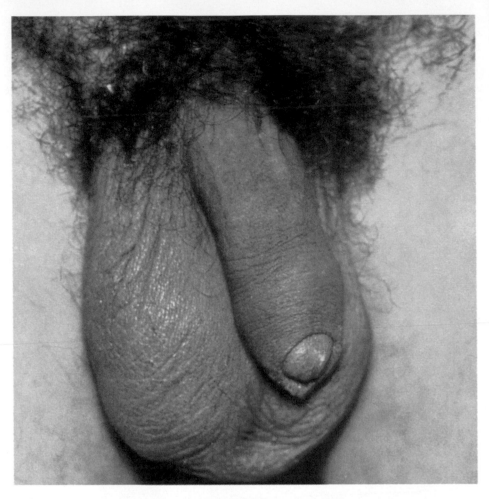

15–1. *Acute epididymitis of right testicle. (Courtesy of Walter E. Stamm, M.D.)*

Patient Profile   Age 28, married electrical engineer

History   Mild left testicular pain beginning 2 days earlier, while playing basketball; increasing pain and swelling for 6 hours; denied urethral discharge and dysuria; sexual intercourse 1 month earlier with a new female sex partner

Examination   Scrotum warm, skin erythematous; testicle indurated, almost twice normal size; marked tenderness, maximal posteriorly, extending into spermatic cord; scant mucoid urethral discharge

Differential Diagnosis   Acute epididymitis; possible trauma, torsion, cancer, tuberculosis, or other granulomatous inflammation

Laboratory   Urethral Gram stain showed >15 PMNs per 1000× (oil immersion) microscopic field, without gram-negative diplococci; leukocyte esterase test on midstream urine (negative); urethral cultures sent for *C. trachomatis* (positive) and *N. gonorrhoeae* (negative); midstream urine culture (no growth)

Diagnosis   Chlamydial epididymitis

Treatment   Ofloxacin 300 mg PO *bid* for 10 days

Partner Management   Advised to refer wife and his new partner for treatment for presumptive chlamydia infection

Other   Counseled about risks associated with unprotected intercourse with unknown partners; condom use advised

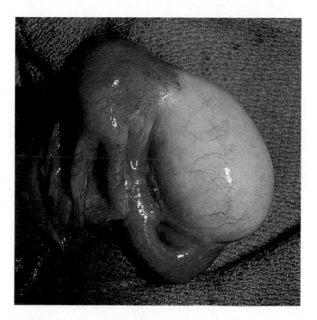

15–2.   *Acute epididymitis due to the antiarrhythmic drug amiodarone; the epididymis is enlarged and erythematous; surgery was performed because tumor was suspected. Infectious epididymitis has a similar appearance. (Courtesy of Richard E. Berger, M.D.)*

ADDITIONAL READING

Berger RE: Acute epididymitis, in *Sexually Transmitted Diseases,* 3d ed. KK Holmes et al (eds). New York, McGraw-Hill, 1999, Chap 61. *A comprehensive review of epididymitis.*

Berger RE et al: Etiology and manifestations of epididymitis in young men: correlations with sexual orientation. *J Infect Dis* 155:1341–1343, 1987. *Report of a consecutive series of young men with epididymitis, documenting high rates of chlamydial and gonococcal infection in heterosexuals and coliform infection in MSM.*

Hoosen AA et al: Microbiology of acute epididymitis in a developing community. *Genitourin Med* 69:361–363, 1993. *A consecutive series in South Africa, documenting frequent chlamydial and gonococcal etiology.*

Chapter 16
REITER'S SYNDROME

Reiter's syndrome is classically described as a triad of urethritis or cervicitis, rheumatoid factor–negative arthritis, and mucocutaneous inflammatory lesions, including conjunctivitis, characteristic dermatitis, and oral mucosal ulcers. Limited forms of Reiter's syndrome, such as "sexually acquired reactive arthritis," are common at presentation, but many such patients eventually develop mucocutaneous or ocular manifestations. Reiter's syndrome is clinically and pathologically related to other reactive spondyloarthropathies, such as ankylosing spondylitis and psoriatic arthritis, and probably results from an aberrant immune response following any of several mucosal infections. Up to 90% of affected persons have the histocompatibility locus A (HLA) B27 haplotype, compared with <10% of the general population. Numerous reports of *Chlamydia trachomatis* antigens, DNA, and occasionally viable organisms in synovial tissues suggest a possibly important role of direct dissemination in the pathogenesis of the syndrome, but the issue is unsettled. Past studies indicated that brief courses of antibiotics do not influence the course of arthritis, but research is underway to determine the efficacy of prolonged antibiotic therapy.

Epidemic Reiter's syndrome often follows shigellosis, yersiniosis, or other enteric infections, whereas sporadic disease usually is triggered by genital infection. Overt epidemics occur primarily in populations with especially high prevalences of the HLA-B27 haplotype, as in Scandinavia, and usually follow outbreaks of enteric infections. In the United States, genital *C. trachomatis* infection is the most common triggering event, but gonorrhea probably triggers some cases, which may present as "postgonococcal arthritis". Pathogenetically, it is possible that Reiter's syndrome is related more directly to mucosal inflammation than to the specific infecting agent. Differentiating Reiter's syndrome from gonococcal arthritis is sometimes difficult, especially in sexually active persons who lack the highly characteristic skin lesions of either syndrome. Some Reiter's syndrome patients become disabled due to chronic arthritis or other complications, but most cases are transient or cause only minor limitations.

EPIDEMIOLOGY

Incidence and Prevalence   Accurate statistics not available; among the most common causes of arthritis in young adults

Transmission   Depends on triggering infection; person-to-person transmission of *Chlamydia*-linked Reiter's syndrome has been reported

Age   Most U.S. cases occur in sexually active age groups; all ages susceptible; cases triggered by enteric infections have occurred in children as well as adults

Sex   Modest male predominance, with male-female ratio 1:1 to 2:1; previously reported male-female ratio as high as 10:1 probably was due in part to reporting bias or underdiagnosis of lower genital tract inflammation in women with seronegative arthritis

Sexual Orientation   No special predilection; MSM may be at increased risk due to sexually acquired enteric infections

Other Risk Factors   Frequency of Reiter's syndrome reported to be 20–35% following chlamydial or enteric infection in persons with HLA-B27 haplotype; HIV-infected persons may be at elevated risk

HISTORY

Incubation Period   Usually 1–4 weeks after onset of trigger infection

Symptoms   Pain, swelling, and limited mobility of joints; usually one to three joints involved in initial episode; most common sites are heel, toes, lumbosacral spine, knee, or ankle, but any joint can be affected; symptoms of urethritis or cervicitis often present; some patients have recent diarrhea or other symptoms of enteric infection; fever and other systemic symptoms usually mild or absent; skin rash, conjunctivitis, and oral ulcers (usually painless) may develop early or late

Epidemiologic History Most patients have behavioral risks for STD or exposure history, or exposure to enteric infection

PHYSICAL EXAMINATION

Trigger Infection Signs of urethritis, cervicitis, or gastrointestinal infection (see Chaps. 14, 17, 20)

Arthritis Inflammatory signs of one or more joints; effusion usually present when large joints involved (e.g., knee, ankle); tenderness often maximal at tendon insertion sites (entheses; Reiter's arthritis sometimes is characterized as an "enthesopathy"); diffuse synovitis of one or more fingers or toes ("sausage digit") is uncommon but classic; often sacroiliac joint tenderness

Mucocutaneous Lesions Characteristic rash is *keratoderma blennorrhagica,* characterized by hyperkeratotic lesions with erythematous base, usually on extremities, sometimes in clusters; often involves palms and soles; resembles psoriasis, both clinically and histologically; may mimic secondary syphilis; pustular component sometimes present; involvement of glans penis in uncircumcised men results in pathognomonic *circinate balanitis;* conjunctivitis often present, usually bilateral; sometimes superficial ulcers of oral mucosa; fever and malaise occasionally present

Other Manifestations Uncommon findings (<1% of cases) include iritis, uveitis, heart block or other cardiac arrhythmias, and focal neurological signs; amyloidosis is rare complication of chronic cases

LABORATORY EVALUATION

No definitive laboratory test; evaluate as for NGU and cervicitis (Chaps. 14, 17), including tests for *C. trachomatis* and *N. gonorrhoeae*; if synovial effusion present, aspirate for bacterial culture, leukocyte count, and analysis for crystals; blood cultures for *N. gonorrhoeae* to exclude dis-seminated gonococcal infection (DGI); if current or recent diarrhea or other gastrointestinal symptoms, test stool for enteric infection, especially *Shigella, Campylobacter,* and *Yersinia*; serum rheumatoid factor test; HLA typing recommended by most authorities; several weeks after onset, x-ray lumbosacral spine, as many cases develop radiological signs of sacroiliitis; erythrocyte sedimentation rate may be useful to follow clinical course and response to therapy

DIAGNOSTIC CRITERIA

The American Rheumatism Association defines Reiter's syndrome as rheumatoid factor–negative arthritis >1 month in duration, associated with urethritis or cervicitis; exclude other causes, especially septic arthritis, DGI, and crystal-induced arthritis; synovial fluid usually has high cell count ($>20,000/\text{mm}^3$) with predominant PMNs; HLA-B27 haplotype helps confirm diagnosis; if DGI or septic arthritis cannot be excluded, failure to respond to antibiotics (unlike DGI or other infectious arthritis) may help establish diagnosis

TREATMENT

Treat trigger infection with appropriate antibiotic, such as azithromycin or doxycycline for chlamydial infection or NGU (Chaps. 2, 14); no evidence that antimicrobial therapy alters course of arthritis or mucocutaneous manifestations, but studies underway to determine effect of prolonged treatment; mainstay of arthritis therapy is indomethacin and other nonsteroidal anti-inflammatory drugs; aspirin and corticosteroids usually ineffective; most patients should be managed in consultation with a rheumatologist

PREVENTION

Manage sex partners and report cases as dictated by triggering infection

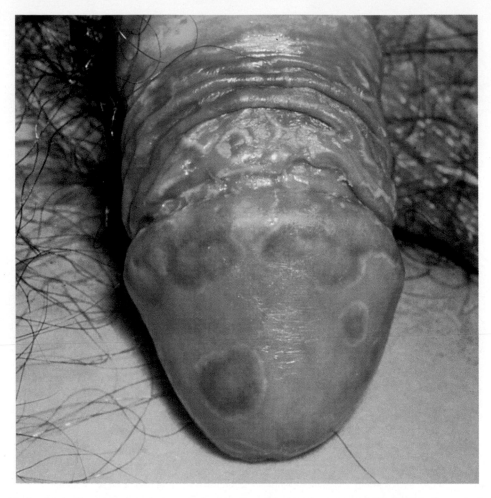

16–1. *Reiter's syndrome: circinate balanitis. (Reprinted with permission from KK Holmes et al (eds),* Sexually Transmitted Diseases, *3d ed. New York, McGraw-Hill, 1999.)*

Patient Profile Age 27, male surgery resident

History Progressive low back pain and intermittent pain in both heels for 4 weeks; rash involving penis and feet for 3 days; pain and swelling of right knee for 1 day; no genital symptoms, diarrhea, fever, or other symptoms; last sexual exposure 2 months previously

Examination Effusion and reduced range of motion of right knee; tenderness at Achilles tendon insertion sites of both heels; "geographic" rash of penis; hyperkeratotic inflammatory skin lesions of lower extremities; no urethral discharge; 50 mL of cloudy synovial fluid aspirated from knee

Differential Diagnosis Reiter's syndrome, psoriatic arthritis, ankylosing spondylitis, rheumatoid arthritis, disseminated gonococcal infection

Laboratory Gram-stained urethral smear showed 10–12 PMNs per 1000× (oil immersion) field, without gram-nagative diplococci; urethral swabs cultured for *C. trachomatis* (positive) and *N. gonorrhoeae* (negative); synovial fluid contained 42,000 leukocytes per mm^3 with 90% PMNs, no crystals, negative Gram stain and culture; rheumatoid factor and VDRL negative; complete blood count and chemistry panel normal; erythrocyte sedimentation rate 43 mm/h; HLA-B27 positive

Diagnosis   Reiter's syndrome

Treatment   Doxycycline 100 mg orally *bid* for 7 days; indomethacin 150 mg orally *tid*

Partner Management   Referred for examination and treatment for chlamydial infection

Comment   Patient had prompt symptomatic response, permitting cessation of indomethacin after 2 months; subsequent chronic but nonlimiting low back pain; sacroiliac radiographs after 1 year showed hypertrophic changes and narrowed joint spaces

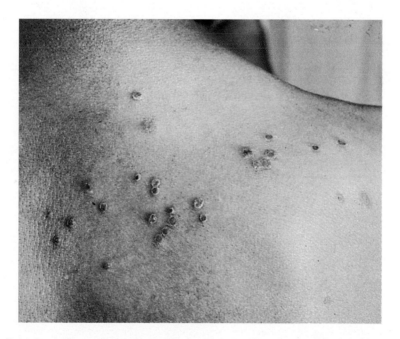

16–2.   *Reiter's syndrome: keratoderma blennorrhagica. (Courtesy of Robert F. Willkens, M.D.)*

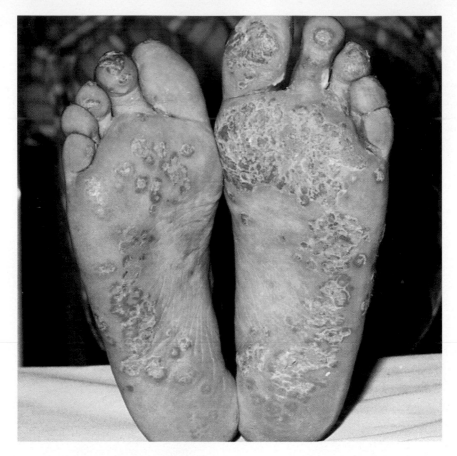

16–3. *Severe plantar keratoderma blennorrhagica in chronic Reiter's syndrome. Compare with secondary syphilis (Fig. 4–15). (Courtesy of Robert F. Willkens, M.D.)*

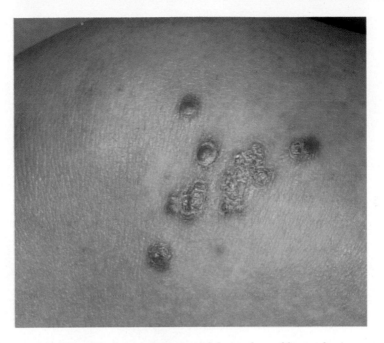

16–4. *Cutaneous lesions of the knee consistent with keratoderma blennorrhagica or psoriasis in a woman with acute spondyloarthritis. The patient was the sex partner of a man with nongonococcal urethritis, but lacked evidence of* Chlamydia trachomatis, *cervicitis, or other lower genital tract infection and was HLA-B27 positive. Reiter's syndrome and psoriatic arthritis could not be differentiated. (Reprinted with permission from KK Holmes et al (eds),* Sexually Transmitted Diseases, *3d ed. New York, McGraw-Hill, 1999.)*

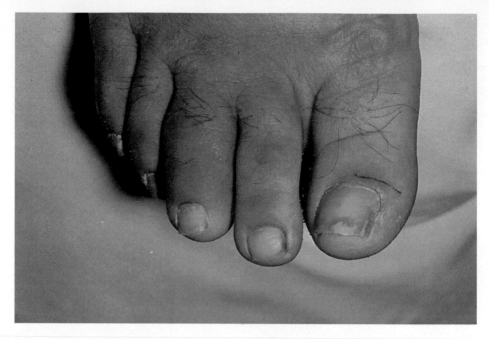

16–5. *Diffuse dactylitis ("sausage toe") of third digit in a patient with Reiter's syndrome. (Courtesy of Robert F. Willkens, M.D.)*

ADDITIONAL READING

Gerard HC et al. Synovial *Chlamydia trachomatis* in patients with reactive arthritis/Reiter's syndrome are viable but show aberrant gene expression. *J Rheumatol* 25:734–742, 1998. *A report of viable* C. trachomatis *from synovial tissues in patients with Reiter's syndrome, with review of the literature.*

Keat AC. Reactive arthritis. *Adv Exp Med Biol* 455:201–206, 1999. *A comprehensive review by a foremost authority, with emphasis on the role of infection in pathogenesis of Reiter's syndrome and related conditions.*

Rice PA, Handsfield HH. Arthritis associated with sexually transmitted diseases, in *Sexually Transmitted Diseases*, 3d ed. KK Holmes et al (eds). New York, McGraw-Hill, 1999, Chap 68. *Review of sexually transmitted arthritis syndromes, especially Reiter's syndrome and disseminated gonococcal infection.*

Chapter 17
MUCOPURULENT CERVICITIS

Mucopurulent cervicitis (MPC) is characterized by inflammation of the endocervical mucosa, as distinguished from ectocervicitis, and is the female counterpart of urethritis in men. The major defined causes are *Chlamydia trachomatis* and *Neisseria gonorrhoeae*, but in common usage MPC usually implies chlamydial or other nongonococcal infection. Herpes simplex virus (HSV) and *Trichomonas vaginalis* cause some cases, usually in conjunction with ectocervicitis. As for urethritis in men, the cause of MPC remains obscure for more than one-half of the cases. Pelvic inflammatory disease is the primary recognized complication but is clearly linked only with chlamydial or gonococcal MPC. Controversy exists about the clinical diagnosis and management of MPC in the absence of gonococcal or chlamydial infection. For example, it is not known whether idiopathic MPC carries important health consequences for the patient or her sex partners, and agreement is lacking on the indications for antibiotic therapy in the absence of chlamydial infection or gonorrhea.

EPIDEMIOLOGY

Incidence and Prevalence Accurate statistics not available; present in 10–30% of women in most STD clinics, but highly variable (in part owing to varying diagnostic criteria)

Transmission As for gonorrhea and chlamydial infection; idiopathic MPC rare in sexually inactive women, implying sexual acquisition or association with intercourse

Age Chlamydial (and probably nonchlamydial) MPC most common in teens (see Chap. 2), perhaps because physiologic cervical ectopy predisposes to MPC

Other Risk Factors Cervical ectopy (i.e., extension of endocervical columnar mucosa onto ectocervix); ectopy may increase risk of infection by exposing an enlarged surface of susceptible epithelium; also, cervical edema may cause partial eversion, exposing endocervical mucosa and creating transient ectopy; hormonal contraception and pregnancy increase risk, probably because they cause ectopy

HISTORY

Incubation Period Poorly studied; probably 1–4 weeks, as for chlamydial infection and gonorrhea

Symptoms Most cases asymptomatic; increased vaginal discharge, usually without malodor; intermenstrual bleeding; postcoital bleeding; dysuria sometimes present due to concomitant urethritis

Epidemiologic History Associated with STD risk factors; especially common in sexually active teens

PHYSICAL EXAMINATION

Mucopurulent exudate emanating from cervical os; purulence (yellow color) of cervical secretions on swab examined outside vagina (positive "swab test"); cervical ectopy with edema of the exposed endocervical mucosa; endocervical bleeding induced by gentle swabbing (sometimes called "friability"); sometimes mild cervical tenderness on bimanual peloric examination

LABORATORY EVALUATION

Gram-stained endocervical smear showing PMNs; absence of PMNs usually excludes MPC, but otherwise no clear consensus on number of PMNs required for diagnosis; observation of PMNs in mucus strands confirms endocervical origin, because vaginal and ectocervical epithelia lack mucus-secreting glands; collect swab specimen carefully to avoid contamination with vaginal secretions; tests for *C. trachomatis* and *N. gonorrhoeae*; microscopic examination for *T. vaginalis* and yeasts (Chaps. 2, 3, 18); test for HSV if history or examination suggests herpes

DIAGNOSIS

Diagnostic Criteria

- Endocervical Gram-stained cervical smear showing increased PMNs, often within strands of mucus; some authorities believe ≥10 PMNs per 1000× microscopic field is abnormal, but others recommend cut-off of ≥30 PMNs per 1000× field; the latter criterion increases specificity for *C. trachomatis* or *N. gonorrhoeae* but reduces sensitivity; PMNs probably normal during menses
- Mucopurulent cervical exudate or positive "swab test"
- Edematous cervical ectopy
- Swab-induced endocervical bleeding

Interpretation Diagnosis normally requires first criterion (increased PMNs) plus at least one other criterion; if microscopic examination not done, presence of ≥2 other criteria usually establishes diagnosis; if only one criterion present, treatment may nonetheless be warranted in presence of other risks for chlamydial infection (e.g., age ≤20 years) or gonorrhea.

MANAGEMENT

Treatment The Centers for Disease Control and Prevention (CDC) advises antimicrobial treatment of MPC only in presence of chlamydial infection, gonorrhea, or specific risk factors for them (e.g., sexual exposure); treat as for uncomplicated chlamydial infection with azithromycin 1.0 g PO (single dose) or doxycycline 100 mg PO *bid* for 7 days (Chap. 2); add single-dose treatment for gonorrhea (Chap. 3) if indicated by risk profile; neither MPC nor any of its manifestations (e.g., edematous ectopy) are indications for cryotherapy, laser cauterization, or other ablative therapies

Follow-Up As for chlamydial infection or gonorrhea (Chaps. 2 and 3); clinical follow-up usually not required unless symptoms persist

PREVENTION

If chlamydial infection or gonorrhea documented or suspected, evaluate and treat sex partners; need for partner treatment uncertain for women with idiopathic MPC (i.e., documented negative tests for *C. trachomatis* and *N. gonorrhoeae*)

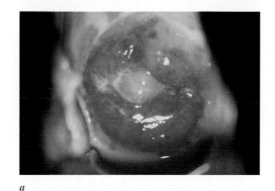

a

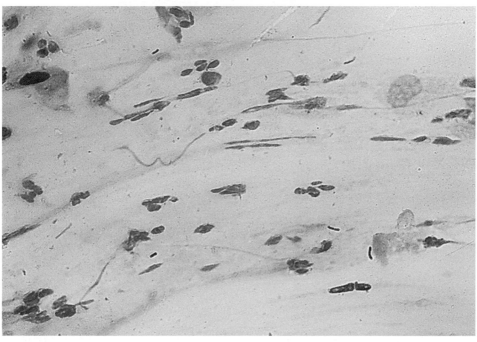

b

17–1. *Mucopurulent cervicitis.* a. *Edematous cervical ectopy and mucopurulent discharge from cervical os.* b. *Gram-stained smear of endocervical secretions, showing PMNs in mucus strands; a few lactobacilli but no gram-negative diplococci are present. Mucus indicates endocervical origin of secretions.*

Patient Profile   Age 16, high school student

History   Slight increased vaginal discharge for 10 days; responded to partner notification after NGU diagnosed in boyfriend

Examination   External genitals normal; cervix showed edematous ectopy, mucopurulent exudate in os

---

Differential Diagnosis   MPC, probably due to *C. trachomatis;* possible gonorrhea, trichomonasis, herpes

Laboratory   Cervical smear showed 10–20 PMNs per 1000× (oil immersion) field, with PMNs in mucus strands, without gram-negative diplococci; vaginal fluid pH 4.0; negative KOH amine odor test; no yeasts, clue cells, or trichomonads seen on wet-mount microscopy; cervical cultures for *C. trachomatis* (positive) and *N. gonorrhoeae* (negative); VDRL, HIV serology (both negative)

Diagnosis   Mucopurulent cervicitis due to *C. trachomatis*

Treatment   Azithromycin 1.0 g PO, single dose

Comment   Typical case of chlamydial MPC; would have qualified for presumptive treatment for chlamydial infection regardless of exposure to infected partner

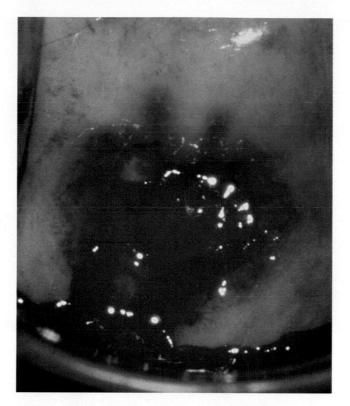

17–2. *Mucopurulent cervicitis; bleeding induced by endocervical swab. (Courtesy of Claire E. Stevens.)*

Patient Profile   Age 33, clerk-receptionist

History   Intermittent increased vaginal discharge without abnormal odor; married 5 years, no extramarital partners; several years' history of intermittent, unexplained vaginal discharge and Pap smears with inflammatory changes

Examination   External genitals normal; cervix showed mucopurulent exudate in os and endocervical bleeding induced by swabs used to collect culture specimens

Differential Diagnosis   Mucopurulent cervicitis (rule out gonorrhea, chlamydial infection), trichomoniasis, herpes

Laboratory   Endocervical smear showed >30 PMNs per 1000× microscopic field; no ICGND; vaginal fluid pH 4.5 with negative KOH amine odor test; no yeasts, clue cells, or trichomonads seen microscopically on wet mount; cervical cultures for *C. trachomatis* and *N. gonorrhoeae* (both negative); VDRL, HIV serology (both negative); Pap smear showed inflammatory cells, otherwise normal

Diagnosis   Idiopathic mucopurulent cervicitis

Treatment   Not treated at initial visit

Comment   Returned in 1 week with persistent symptoms and unchanged examination; husband examined and found to have no evidence of urethritis, negative tests for *C. trachomatis* and *N. gonorrhoeae,* denied other partners; patient treated with doxycycline 100 mg PO *bid* for 7 days; after discussing uncertain need for partner treatment and likelihood of no benefit, patient and husband elected for him to be treated with doxycycline; symptoms persisted on therapy, then improved over next 2 months, but repeat examination unchanged; typical case of idiopathic MPC, without clear evidence of sexual acquisition or therapeutic effect of doxycycline

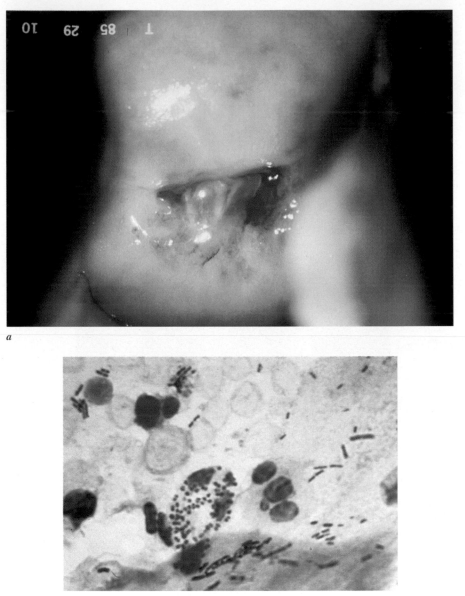

17–3. *Mucopurulent cervicitis due to* Neisseria gonorrhoeae. a. *Mucoid endocervical exudate; mucoid rather than overtly purulent exudate may be seen in gonococcal cervicitis. (Compare with Figs 2–2, 3–2, and 17–1a.)* b. *Gram-stained endocervical smear, showing a single PMN with ICGND. (Courtesy of Claire E. Stevens.)*

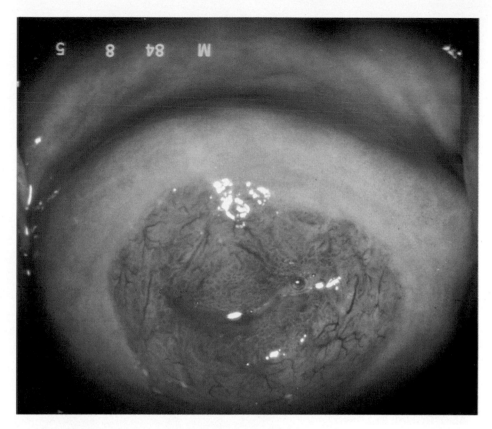

17–4. *Mucopurulent cervicitis due to* Chlamydia trachomatis; *edematous cervical ectopy and scant mucoid exudate. (Courtesy of Claire E. Stevens.)*

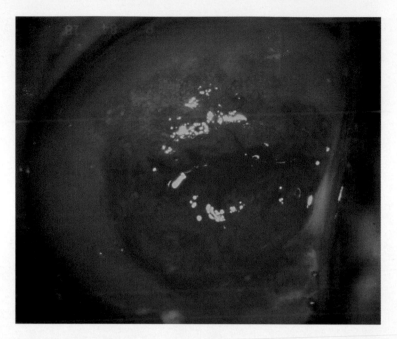

17–5. *Edematous ectopy with incipient endocervical bleeding in a patient with mucopurulent cervicitis; her chief complaint was postcoital bleeding. (Courtesy of Claire E. Stevens.)*

ADDITIONAL READING

Brunham RC et al: Mucopurulent cervicitis: the ignored counterpart in women of urethritis in men. *N Engl J Med* 311:1–6, 1984. *The first systematic description of the clinical syndrome and etiology, still clinically applicable.*

Holmes KK, Stamm WE: Lower genital tract infection syndromes in women, in *Sexually Transmitted Diseases*, 3d ed. KK Holmes et al (eds). New York, McGraw-Hill, 1999, Chap 57. *An authoritative, comprehensive review of cervical, urethral, and urinary tract infections in women.*

Ryan CA et al. Risk assessment, symptoms and signs as predictors of vulvovaginal and cervical infections in an urban U.S. STD clinic: implications for the use of STD algorithms. *Sex Transm Infect* 74 (Suppl 1):S59–S76, 1998. *An analysis of lower genital tract symptoms and signs, with behavioral, diagnostic, and clinical correlations in 779 consecutive women in the Seattle STD Clinic.*

Chapter 18
VAGINAL INFECTIONS

Vulvovaginal yeast infections, bacterial vaginosis, and trichomoniasis are among the most common reasons for which women seek health care. All sexually active women with trichomoniasis or new onset of bacterial vaginosis, and many with candidiasis, should be evaluated for common STDs.

Vulvovaginal candidiasis (VVC) generally is not sexually transmitted, although infections occasionally are acquired from partners with genital or oral colonization. *Candida albicans, Candida* (formerly *Torulopsis*) *glabrata,* and a few other species of yeasts commonly colonize the vagina, and a variety of known factors (e.g., suppression of vaginal bacterial flora by antibiotics) and unknown ones result in proliferation of these organisms or development of an allergic response to them. Symptomatic VVC typically is accompanied by symptoms and signs of vulvitis, often a helpful diagnostic feature, yet vaginal fluid leukocytosis usually is absent. Effective vaginal preparations for treatment of VVC are available over the counter without prescription, but undoubtedly are used inappropriately by many women who have other causes of vaginal discharge or vulvar pruritus. The use of these products should be discouraged except in women with classic symptoms who have previously had a professional diagnosis of VVC.

Bacterial vaginosis (BV) is characterized by absence of facultative *Lactobacillus* sp. in the vagina and overgrowth of commensal vaginal bacteria, including *Gardnerella vaginalis, Mobiluncus* sp., *Mycoplasma hominis,* and numerous anaerobes. Depletion of hydrogen peroxide–producing lactobacilli appears to be the initial pathologic event, but the specific causes are unknown. No sexually transmitted pathogen has been found, and treatment of women's male partners does not influence the rate of recurrence following treatment of BV. Nevertheless, BV is associated with sexual intercourse and with epidemiologic markers for STD, such as multiple sex partners, new partners, and past history of STDs, and direct sexual transmission of BV apparently occurs in women who have sex with women (WSW) through exchange of vaginal secretions. There is little or no inflammatory response and leukocytes usually are not found in vaginal fluid, hence the term *vaginosis,* not vaginitis. Bacterial vaginosis is associated with increased risk of pelvic inflammatory disease (PID), premature labor, and other complications of labor and delivery, although the frequency of adverse pregnancy outcomes apparently is not reduced by treatment of BV during pregnancy. Many women with BV attempt self-treatment with vaginal douching, probably because they believe odor implies a hygiene problem. However, vaginal douching itself predisposes to BV and is strongly linked with increased risk of PID and ectopic pregnancy. Douching for any reason, including vulvovaginal "hygiene," odor, discharge, or following menstruation or intercourse, should be strongly discouraged.

Trichomoniasis is an extremely common sexually transmitted infection caused by the unicellular parasite *Trichomonas vaginalis.* Most apparent exceptions to sexual transmission are explained by delayed diagnosis of longstanding infection, and some monogamous women are infected by chronically infected partners. Symptomatic trichomoniasis is associated with an inflammatory response and vaginal leukocytosis. Anaerobic bacterial overgrowth and depletion of lactobacilli often occur, as in BV. Other STDs are often present in young women with recently acquired trichomoniasis. Single-dose treatment with oral metronidazole is highly effective, although slightly less so than multiple-dose therapy; topical therapy is ineffective.

Uncommon causes of vulvovaginal infection or increased vaginal discharge include retained foreign bodies (e.g., tampons), enterovaginal fistulas, and estrogen deficiency. Physiologic fluctuations in the quantity or character of cervicovaginal secretions explain some women's complaints of increased vaginal discharge.

EPIDEMIOLOGY

Incidence and Prevalence All three syndromes extremely common in young women, but reliable statistics not available; among women attending STD or reproductive health clinics, VVC is diagnosed in 20–25%, BV in 10–20%, trichomoniasis in 5–15%

Transmission Vaginal colonization with *Candida* and other yeasts often originates from colonic reservoir; transmission of BV uncertain, associated with sexual activity; in WSW, BV apparently directly transmitted by vaginal secretions; *T. vaginalis* is sexually acquired, with few if any exceptions

Age All ages susceptible; most common in sexually active young women; trichomoniasis in older women sometimes due to delayed diagnosis of chronic infection

Sex No known male counterpart to BV; male partners of women with VVC sometimes have penile *Candida* dermatitis or balanitis; *T. vaginalis* colonizes male urethra and periurethral glands, usually without symptoms, but sometimes causes NGU

Sexual Orientation BV common in WSW, probably sexually acquired; WSW not obviously at either increased or decreased risk for VVC or trichomoniasis, but few data available

Douching and Contraception Douching, diaphragm, contraceptive sponge, and other nonoxynol-9–containing creams or foams apparently predispose to BV and perhaps VVC

Other Risk Factors Antibiotic therapy predisposes to VVC and probably BV; poorly controlled diabetes mellitus predisposes to vaginal colonization with *Candida*, but diabetes rarely found in young women with recurrent VVC; HIV infection not associated with substantially enhanced risk of VVC, despite earlier reports to the contrary; however, HIV infection may impair response to therapy; notwithstanding common beliefs, tight-fitting garments probably do not predispose to VVC

HISTORY

Incubation Period Highly variable; symptoms of trichomoniasis or BV often begin a few days to 4 weeks after exposure to new or recently infected sex partner

Symptoms

VULVOVAGINAL CANDIDIASIS Vulvar burning pain or pruritus; "external" dysuria due to urine contacting inflamed introitus and labia; vaginal discharge usually absent or scant; usually no malodor (contrary to popular belief)

BACTERIAL VAGINOSIS Genital malodor, often described as "fishy," is most common symptom; odor may be more prominent following intercouse, because alkaline semen volatilizes amines; increased vaginal discharge, usually without prominent staining of underclothes; often asymptomatic

TRICHOMONIASIS Increased vaginal discharge, often profuse; staining of underclothes; sometimes malodor; sometimes vulvar pruritus

Epidemiologic History Risk factors for STD often present in women with BV or trichomoniasis; history of vaginal douching common in women with BV and perhaps VVC; antibiotic use precedes some yeast infections and BV; women with BV or VVC often give history of previous vulvovaginal infections

PHYSICAL EXAMINATION

Vulvovaginal Candidiasis Vulvar erythema, sometimes with edema or superficial fissures; typical discharge is scant, clumped, white, adherent to vaginal mucosa; however, homogeneous, flocculant, or purulent-appearing exudate sometimes seen

Bacterial Vaginosis Usually scant to moderate discharge; usually white, homogeneous, smoothly coating vaginal walls or labia; usually no erythema or other inflammatory signs

Trichomoniasis Homogeneous discharge, often copious; usually purulent (yellow); sometimes mucosal erythema; occasional petechiae on ectocervix ("colpitis macularis," "strawberry cervix"); bubbles in vaginal fluid are classic and highly specific for trichomoniasis, but usually not seen

DIAGNOSTIC APPROACH

The first step in evaluating a woman with vaginal discharge or other vulvovaginal complaints is a speculum examination to determine whether abnormal secretions originate from the vagina or cervix. The character of the vaginal discharge is assessed and the vaginal mucosa and vulva are inspected for erythema, edema, ulcers, and other lesions. Determination of the pH of vaginal abnormal secretions, the presence or absence of fishy amine odors on addition of a few drops of 10% KOH, together with microscopic examination (by wet mount, Gram stain, or both) of vaginal secretions usually permit an accurate office diagnosis. Cultures for *T. vaginalis* and yeasts often are helpful if the diagnosis remains obscure. If microscopy is not readily available, such cultures assume greater importance; rapid, office-based immunochemical tests for BV (e.g., based on semiquantitation of *G. vaginalis*) may also be useful. Screening tests for chlamydial infection, gonorrhea, syphilis, and HIV infection should be routine in all women with trichomoniasis, most with initial episodes of BV, and selected women with VVC, depending on sexual history.*

LABORATORY DIAGNOSIS

Vulvovaginal Candidiasis Vaginal fluid pH ≤4.5; negative amine odor with 10% KOH; vaginal fluid microscopy (Gram-stained smear or saline mount) demonstrates pseudohyphae or yeasts in ~80% of patients; visualization of yeasts alone (without pseudohyphae) may indicate colonization only; PMNs usually scant or absent; KOH wet mount highlights fungal elements because KOH digests cells and mucus; isolation of *Candida* helpful if microscopy negative, but may be positive owing to colonization not related to vaginitis

Bacterial Vaginosis Vaginal fluid pH ≥4.7; amine ("fishy") odor with 10% KOH (liberates volatile amines produced by anaerobic bacteria); saline mount or Gram-stained smear shows clue cells (epithelial cells with indistinct borders and granular appearance due to adherent bacteria); usually no PMNs; Gram stain shows clue cells and profusion of mixed gram-positive and gram-negative bacteria, and absence of large gram-positive bacilli typical of *Lactobacillus* sp.

Trichomoniasis Vaginal fluid pH ≥5.0; motile trichomonads and predominant PMNs on microscopy of vaginal fluid mixed with normal saline; if trichomonads not seen, culture for *T. vaginalis* is useful; often clue cells and positive amine odor test; saline mount or Gram-stained

smear often shows changes in bacterial flora similar to BV

TREATMENT

Vulvovaginal Candidiasis

ACUTE INFECTION

- Fluconazole 150–200 mg PO (single dose)
- Any of several imidazole creams or suppositories (butoconazole, clotrimazole, econazole, miconazole, terconazole, tioconazole), usually administered once daily for 3–7 days; single-dose regimens not recommended

PREVENTION OF RECURRENT INFECTION

- Antifungal therapy to prevent recurrences indicated in some women with frequently recurring infection
- Fluconazole 100 mg PO once weekly
- Clotrimazole 500 mg intravaginally once weekly

Bacterial Vaginosis

TREATMENT OF CHOICE

- Metronidazole 500 mg PO *bid* for 7 days

ALTERNATIVES

- Metronidazole 2.0 g PO, single dose, when compliance with multiple-dose therapy is unlikely; higher relapse rate than with multiple-dose therapy
- Metronidazole 0.75% gel, 5 g intravaginally daily or *bid* for 5 days
- Clindamycin 2% cream, 5 g intravaginally *qd* for 7 days
- Clindamycin 300 mg PO *bid* for 7 days; probably higher relapse rate because clindamycin is active against *Lactobacillus* sp. and may interfere with reestablishment of normal flora

COMMENT Do not prescribe (and assertively discourage) vaginal douching for treatment or prevention; topical or systemic sulfonamides, tetracyclines, and other antibiotics are ineffective systemically or topically; currently available *Lactobacillus* preparations and dairy products (e.g., yogurt) do not contain physiologic *Lactobacillus* strains that produce hydrogen peroxide, do not successfully colonize the vagina, and are ineffective for treatment or prophylaxis, whether used orally or intravaginally; promis-

*See Table 18–1 on page 166 for a listing of the diagnostic features of vaginal infection in premenopausal women.

Table 18–1   DIAGNOSTIC FEATURES OF VAGINAL INFECTION IN PREMENOPAUSAL WOMEN

	NORMAL	YEAST VULVOVAGINITIS	TRICHOMONAL VAGINITIS	BACTERIAL VAGINOSIS
Typical symptoms	None	Vulvar itching and/or irritation; sometimes increased discharge	Purulent discharge, often profuse; sometimes vulvar pruritus	Vulvovaginal malodor; slightly increased discharge
Discharge				
Amount	Variable; usually scant	Scant to moderate	Profuse	Scant to moderate
Color*	Clear or white	White or yellow	Yellow, tan	Usually white
Consistency	Nonhomogeneous, floccular	Clumped; adherent plaques	Homogeneous	Homogeneous, low viscosity; smoothly coats vaginal mucosa
Inflammation of vulvar or vaginal epithelium	None	Erythema of vaginal epithelium, introitus; vulvar dermatitis common	Erythema of vaginal and vulvar epithelium; sometimes petechiae of ectocervix ("strawberry cervix")	None
pH of vaginal fluid†	Usually ≤4.5	Usually ≤4.5	Usually ≥5.0	Usually ≥4.7
Amine (fishy) odor with 10% KOH	None	None	Present	Present
Microscopy‡	Normal epithelial cells; lactobacilli predominate (large gram-positive rods)	Epithelial cells; yeasts or pseudomycelia (up to 80%); usually few PMNs	PMNs; motile trichomonads in 80–90% of symptomatic patients, less often in absence of symptoms	Clue cells; profuse mixed flora with few or no lactobacilli

*Color of discharge is best determined by examining discharge outside vagina against a white background.
†pH determination is not useful if blood is present.
‡To detect fungal elements, vaginal fluid is digested with 10% KOH prior to microscopic examination; to examine for other features, fluid is mixed (1:1) with physiologic saline. Gram stain also is excellent for detecting yeasts and pseudomycelia and for distinguishing normal flora from the mixed flora seen in bacterial vaginosis, but is insensitive for detection of *T. vaginalis.*

ing research underway with appropriate *Lacto-bacillus* strains to restore physiologic flora

Trichomoniasis

- Metronidazole 2.0 g PO, single dose
- Metronidazole 500 mg PO *bid* for 7 days,[†] if single-dose treatment fails

Sex Partner Management

VULVOVAGINAL CANDIDIASIS Partner examination or treatment usually not indicated; if history suggests penile dermatitis, treat with an imidazole cream

BACTERIAL VAGINOSIS Partner examination optional, depending on STD risk; usually evaluate male partners of women with first-episode BV, especially if new or multiple partners; routine treatment of partners for BV not indicated; advise WSW of risk of BV in partners

TRICHOMONIASIS Evaluate partners for urethritis and other STD; treat routinely with metronidazole 2.0 g PO (single dose)

[†]A new preparation of 375 mg metronidazole, administered *bid,* appears to be effective and probably is a suitable alternative regimen, but it is not available generically and experience is limited.

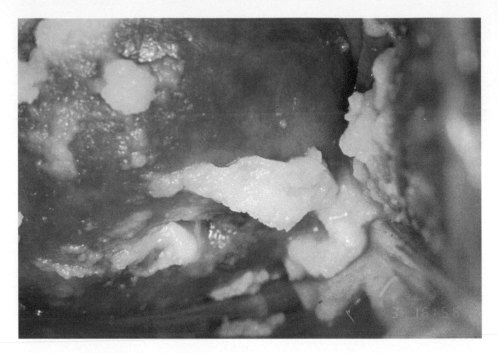

18–1. *Clumped vaginal exudate in vulvovaginitis due to* Candida albicans. *(Courtesy of Claire E. Stevens.)*

Patient Profile   Age 20, college student, sexually active with one male partner

History   Vulvar itching and slightly increased vaginal discharge for 2 days

Examination   Erythema of vaginal mucosa and labia; clumped white discharge in plaques on vaginal mucosa and cervix; otherwise normal

Differential Diagnosis   Vulvovaginal candidiasis; trichomoniasis, BV, and MPC less likely

Laboratory   Vaginal fluid pH 4.0; amine odor test negative; microscopic examination showed yeasts and pseudohyphae; cervical LCR test for *C. trachomatis* (negative)

Diagnosis   Vulvovaginal candidiasis

Treatment   Fluconazole 150 mg PO (single dose)

Management of Sex Partner   Patient advised to ascertain that partner has no penile rash or other genital symptoms

Other   Screening test for *C. trachomatis* obtained on the basis of age ≤20 years; tests for other STDs optional

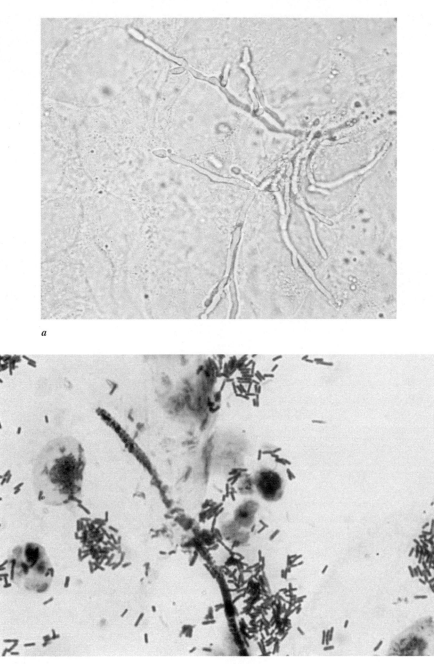

a

b

18–2. *Microscopic findings in vulvovaginal candidiasis.* a. *Potassium hydroxide digest of vaginal secretions, showing pseudohyphae of* Candida albicans. *(Courtesy of David A. Eschenbach, M.D.)* b. *Gram-stained smear of vaginal secretions, showing typically mottled, gram-positive pseudohypha of* Candida albicans *and multiple* Lactobacillus *morphotypes. (Courtesy of Sharon L. Hillier, Ph.D.)*

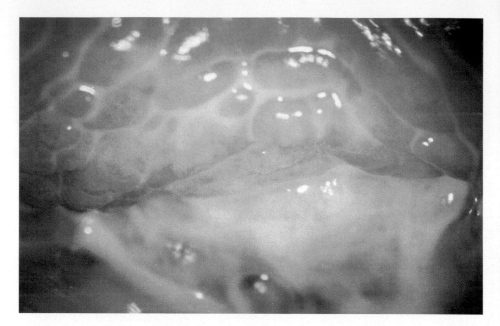

18–3. *Bacterial vaginosis; white, homogeneous discharge smoothly coating the vaginal mucosa. Also see Fig. 9–2. (Courtesy of Claire E. Stevens.)*

Patient Profile   Age 22, single, photographer's assistant

History   Increased vaginal discharge with a "strong" odor for 1 week, especially after sex; one male partner in a relationship that began 1 month previously; past history of chlamydial infection and genital warts

Examination   Homogeneous white vaginal secretions at introitus and coating vaginal mucosa; cervix showed small area of ectopy, with slightly cloudy mucus in os; bimanual examination normal

Differential Diagnosis   Probable bacterial vaginosis; consider trichomoniasis, vulvovaginal candidiasis, chlamydial cervicitis, gonorrhea, physiologic discharge

Laboratory   Vaginal fluid pH 5.0; amine odor with addition of 10% KOH; saline wet-mount microscopy showed clue cells, no trichomonads, rare PMNs; cervical swab specimens for *C. trachomatis* and *N. gonorrhoeae*, VDRL, HIV serology (all negative)

Diagnosis   Bacterial vaginosis

Treatment   Metronidazole 500 mg PO *bid* for 7 days

Partner Management   Advised to refer her partner for STD evaluation to exclude other STDs; treatment of partner for BV not indicated

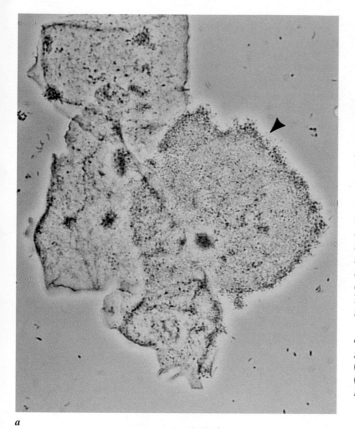

18–4. *Microscopic findings in bacterial vaginosis. a. Clue cell (arrow) adjacent to normal vaginal epithelial cells; the clue cell has an indistinct, ragged margin and a refractile, granular appearance due to large numbers of adherent bacteria. (Courtesy of David A. Eschenbach, M.D.) b. Gram-stained smears of secretions in bacterial vaginosis (left) and normal vaginal secretions (right); the bacterial vaginosis smear shows numerous small, pleomorphic, gram-negative and gram-positive bacteria that heavily coat a clue cell and absence of* Lactobacillus *morphotypes; the normal smear shows "clean" epithelial cells and predominant large, gram-positive bacilli (*Lactobacillus *sp.). (Courtesy of Sharon L. Hillier, Ph.D.)*

a

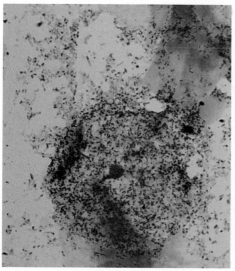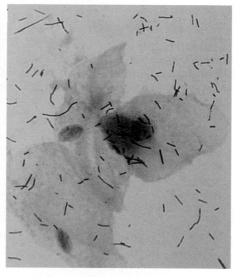

b

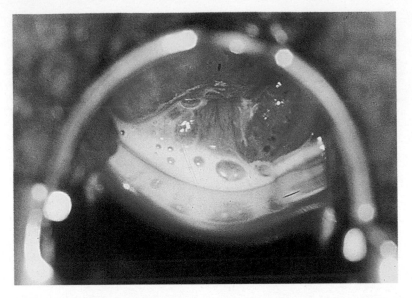

18–5. *Purulent vaginal discharge in trichomonal vaginitis; bubbles due to gas production by anaerobic bacteria are seen in a minority of cases, but are highly specific for trichomoniasis; mucopurulent cervical discharge and edematous cervical ectopy also are present.*

Patient Profile   Age 24, single, unemployed woman, referred from a drug rehabilitation agency

History   Increased vaginal discharge and slight vulvar pruritus for 2 weeks; one male partner for 6 months

Examination   External genitals normal; copious, malodorous, faintly yellow vaginal discharge with bubbles; cervical ectopy and mucopurulent cervical discharge; no adnexal tenderness or masses

Differential Diagnosis   Trichomoniasis, bacterial vaginosis; rule out vulvovaginal candidiasis, gonorrhea, chlamydial infection

Laboratory   Vaginal fluid pH 5.5; amine odor test positive; saline preparation showed PMNs, motile trichomonads, few clue cells; endocervical Gram stain showed 20 PMNs per 1000× field, without gram-negative diplococci; cultures for *C. trachomatis* (negative) and *N. gonorrhoeae* (positive); VDRL (negative); HIV serology (positive)

Diagnosis   Trichomonal vaginitis; gonorrhea; HIV infection

Treatment   Metronidazole 2.0 g PO (single dose); patient called back after *N. gonorrhoeae* isolated and given cefixime 400 mg PO and azithromycin 1.0 g PO (both single dose)

Partner Management   Partner contacted; treated with metronidazole, cefixime, and azithromycin; also found to be HIV-positive

Comment   Trichomoniasis often is associated with other STDs, such as gonorrhea; previously unknown HIV infection diagnosed; patient and partner referred for HIV/AIDS evaluation and care

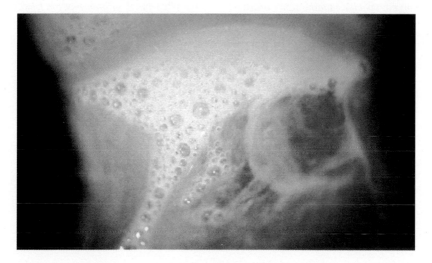

18–6. *Saline of vaginal secretions in trichomoniasis, showing two* T. vaginalis *(arrows) and leukocytes; in actual use, trichomonads are readily distinguished from leukocytes by their motility.*

18–7. *Frothy vaginal discharge in trichomonal vaginitis. (Courtesy of Claire E. Stevens.)*

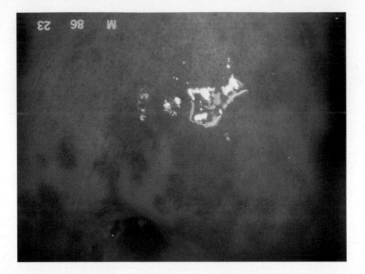

18–8. *Cervical petechiae, sometimes called "colpitis macularis" or "strawberry cervix," an uncommon but specific manifestation of trichomoniasis. (Reprinted with permission from KK Holmes et al (eds),* Sexually Transmitted Diseases, *3d ed. New York, McGraw-Hill, 1999.)*

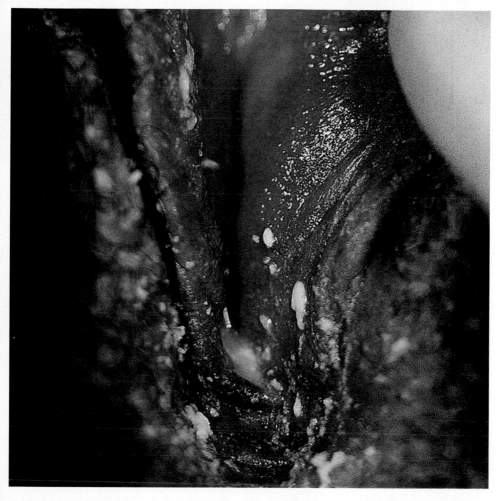

18–9. *Candida vulvovaginitis; erythema of labia minora and scant, clumped white exudate.*

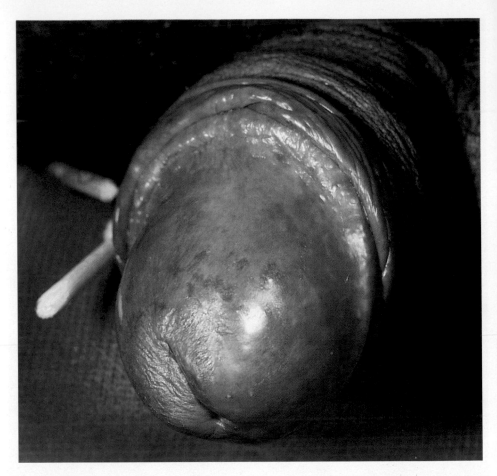

18–10. *Balanitis due to* Candida albicans; *punctate lesions of glans penis in the uncircumcised partner of a woman with vulvovaginal candidiasis.*

ADDITIONAL READING

Carey JC et al: Metronidazole to prevent preterm delivery in pregnant women with asymptomatic bacterial vaginosis. *N Engl J Med* 342:534–540, 2000. *Report of a prospective study, showing that despite the association of BV with preterm labor and delivery, treatment did not affect outcome. An excellent entry to the literature on vaginal infections and pregnancy outcome.*

Hillier S, Holmes KK: Bacterial vaginosis, in *Sexually Transmitted Diseases,* 3d ed, KK Holmes et al (eds). New York, McGraw-Hill, 1999, Chap 42. *A comprehensive overview of pathogenesis, epidemiology, and clinical manifestations.*

Holmes KK, Stamm WE: Lower genital tract infection syndromes in women, in *Sexually Transmitted Diseases,* 3d ed, KK Holmes et al (eds). New York, McGraw-Hill, 1999, Chap 57. *An overview of lower genital tract infections in women, including differential diagnosis of vaginal discharge and other vulvovaginal symptoms.*

Krieger JN, Alderete JF: *Trichomonas vaginalis* and trichomoniasis, in *Sexually Transmitted Diseases,* 3d ed, KK Holmes et al (eds). New York, McGraw-Hill, 1999, Chap 43. *A comprehensive overview of pathogenesis, epidemiology, and clinical manifestations of trichomoniasis.*

Krieger JN: Trichomoniasis in men: old issues and new data. *Sex Transm Dis* 22:83–96, 1995. *An overview of the clinical manifestations, diagnosis, and treatment of the male component of trichomoniasis.*

Sobel JD: Vulvovaginal candidiasis in *Sexually Transmitted Diseases,* 3d ed, KK Holmes et al (eds). New York, McGraw-Hill, 1999, Chap 45. *A comprehensive overview of pathogenesis, epidemiology, and clinical manifestations of VVC.*

Sobel JD et al: Single-dose fluconazole compared with conventional clotrimazole topical therapy of *Candida vaginitis. Am J Obstet Gynecol* 172:1263–1268, 1995. *A randomized controlled trial documenting the efficacy of single-dose oral fluconazole for VVC.*

Zhang J et al: Vaginal douching and adverse health effects: a meta-analysis. *Am J Pub Health* 87:1207–1211, 1997. *Review of published literature, confirming the strong association of vaginal douching with STDs, pelvic inflammatory disease, and ectopic pregnancy.*

Chapter 19
PELVIC INFLAMMATORY DISEASE

Pelvic inflammatory disease (PID) is the most common serious STD complication. PID is defined as salpingitis, often accompanied by endometritis or secondary pelvic peritonitis, that results from ascending genital infection that is unrelated to childbirth or surgical manipulation. At least 90% of cases meeting these criteria are sexually acquired, but a few cases are attributed to ascending infection with nonsexually transmitted organisms. The main sequelae of PID are infertility and ectopic pregnancy that result from tubal scarring. The risk of infertility following symptomatic PID is estimated to be 15–20%, but this varies with the causative agent, the severity of PID as documented by laparoscopy, and the number of PID episodes. A past history of PID enhances the risk of subsequent episodes, probably because scarring impairs normal tubal clearance mechanisms. Although PID is sometimes clinically severe, accompanied by fever, tubo-ovarian abscess, peritonitis, and other systemic manifestations, most cases are mild; indeed, subclinical salpingitis is estimated to account for 60% of all cases, and most women with tubal-factor infertility or ectopic pregnancy have no past history of PID or unexplained abdominal pain. "Chronic" PID is an indistinct entity; the term sometimes is used inappropriately for pelvic adhesions and unexplained pelvic pain, without evidence of infection or active inflammation.

Chlamydia trachomatis is the most common cause of acute PID in industrialized countries and the likely cause of most subclinical cases. *Neisseria gonorrhoeae* remains a major cause where gonorrhea remains common. Numerous other bacteria contribute to PID, including *Mycoplasma hominis* and various aerobic and anaerobic components of the vaginal flora, and most women with acute PID have signs of bacterial vaginosis (BV). It is probable that any of several inflammatory events involving the endocervix, such as gonorrhea, chlamydial infection, and perhaps nonchlamydial cervicitis or BV, may result in ascending endometrial and tubal infection with the primary pathogen, vaginal bacteria, or both. Rarely, a nonsexually transmitted pathogen (e.g., *Haemophilus influenzae*) is isolated in pure culture from the fallopian tubes or culdocentesis aspirate, suggesting that not all cases of PID are sexually acquired. The specific bacteria contributing to salpingitis usually are not known in individual patients, and treatment for acute PID must be adequate for gonorrhea, chlamydial infection, and mixed aerobic and anaerobic flora.

EPIDEMIOLOGY

Incidence and Prevalence   Estimated 600,000 to 1 million cases annually in the United States; diagnosed in 1–5% of women in U.S. STD clinics; overt or subclinical PID is the most common cause of ectopic pregnancy and tubal infertility; 70–80% of women with tubal infertility or ectopic pregnancy are *C. trachomatis*-seropositive, compared with 30–40% with nontubal infertility

Transmission   As for *C. trachomatis* and *N. gonorrhoeae* (Chaps. 2, 3)

Age   Risk rises with decreasing age in sexually active women; markedly increased risk in sexually active teens, probably due to both behavioral and physiologic factors (e.g., susceptibility to *C. trachomatis* and *N. gonorrhoeae*)

Sexual Orientation   Probably uncommon in women who have sex only with women

Other Risk Factors   Vaginal douching markedly increases risk of PID and ectopic pregnancy, behavioral markers of STD risk; intrauterine device (IUD) for contraception; previous PID; repeated chlamydial infection; hormonal contraception apparently reduces risk of symptomatic chlamydial PID; HIV infection may increase risk and perhaps severity of PID

HISTORY

Incubation Period   Varies from 1–2 days to several months following acquisition of *C. trachomatis* or *N. gonorrhoeae*

Symptoms   Most cases mild or subclinical; low abdominal pain nearly universal in symptomatic cases; most patients have vaginal discharge or other symptoms of MPC or BV (Chaps. 17, 18); often dyspareunia, menorrhagia, intermenstrual bleeding, sometimes right upper quadrant abdominal pain; fever, chills, malaise, nausea, and vomiting suggest severe infection

Epidemiologic History   Often young age, especially <25 years; usually new sex partner or other STD risks

PHYSICAL EXAMINATION

Pelvic adnexal tenderness, usually bilateral, of variable severity; uterine fundal and cervical motion tenderness; usually signs of MPC or BV; fever common but often absent; palpable adnexal mass sometimes present; lower quadrant abdominal tenderness, sometimes with rebound tenderness or other peritoneal inflammatory signs; sometimes right upper quadrant tenderness due to perihepatitis (Fitz-Hugh–Curtis syndrome), especially with chlamydial PID

LABORATORY DIAGNOSIS

Lower Genital Tract Infection   Usually laboratory evidence of MPC, BV, or both (see Chaps. 17 and 18)

Microbiology   Endocervical tests for *N. gonorrhoeae* and *C. trachomatis;* if laparoscopy done, test tubal aspirate or peritoneal exudate for *N. gonorrhoeae* and *C. trachomatis* and culture for aerobic and anaerobic bacteria

Other Tests   Leukocyte count and either erythrocyte sedimentation rate (ESR) or assay for C-reactive protein should be performed (indicators of clinical severity, but normal results do not exclude PID); pelvic ultrasound examination sometimes helpful; laparoscopy indicated in severe cases if diagnosis uncertain or if inadequate response to antibiotics; endome-

trial biopsy can be helpful in documenting endometritis, which is usually present in PID; recommend HIV testing for all patients

DIAGNOSTIC CRITERIA

In young sexually active women, low abdominal pain plus adnexal or cervical motion tenderness indicate sufficient likelihood of PID to warrant presumptive treatment; specificity of diagnosis rises with documentation of gonococcal or chlamydial infection and with elevated leukocyte count, ESR, or C-reactive protein; only two-thirds of patients with clinically diagnosed PID have laparoscopic evidence of salpingitis; severity of PID as documented by laparoscopy correlates poorly with severity of clinical symptoms and signs

TREATMENT

Principles   Treat all suspected cases while awaiting diagnostic confirmation; routinely cover *N. gonorrhoeae, C. trachomatis,* and mixed aerobic and anaerobic bacteria, regardless of pathogens identified in patient or sex partner or apparent clinical severity; short-term clinical efficacy is similar for all recommended regimens, but efficacies unknown for preservation of fertility; indications for hospitalization or parenteral therapy are possible surgical emergency (e.g., appendicitis), pregnancy, severe manifestations (e.g., nausea, vomiting, high fever, peritonitis), poor response to oral therapy, suspected tubo-ovarian abscess, or inability to follow oral regimen

Recommended Regimens

INPATIENT TREATMENT   Use regimen A for probable chlamydial or gonococcal PID; regimen B preferred by some experts when predominant aerobic and anaerobic infection is likely (e.g., recurrent PID or IUD-related PID in a woman at low risk for STD)

- *Regimen A*: Doxycycline 100 mg IV or PO* every 12 h, plus either cefotetan 2.0 g IV every 12 h or cefoxitin 2.0 g IV every 6 h; continue until clinical improvement begins (at least 48 h), then give doxycycline 100 mg PO *bid* to complete 14 days total therapy.

*Doxycycline administered IV or PO provides similar blood levels; oral therapy may be used if tolerated

- *Regimen B*: Clindamycin 900 mg IV every 8 h, plus gentamicin, 2.0 mg/kg body weight (loading dose), then 1.5 mg/kg every 8 h (or an equivalent single-dose daily regimen); continue both until clinical improvement seen (at least 48 h), then give doxycycline 100 mg PO *bid*, or clindamycin 450 mg PO *qid,* or both, to complete 14 days total therapy.
- *Alternative parenteral regimens*: Other regimens, providing coverage for all likely pathogens but less completely studied, are ofloxacin 400 mg IV every 12 h, plus metronidazole 500 mg IV every 8 h; ampicillin/sulbactam 3 g IV every 6 h, plus doxycycline 100 mg IV or PO every 12 h; and ciprofloxacin 200 mg IV every 12 h, plus doxycycline 100 mg IV or PO every 12 h, plus metronidazole 500 mg IV every 8 h

OUTPATIENT TREATMENT   Two alternative regimens recommended; regimen A provides superior coverage for anaerobic bacteria but is more expensive than regimen B

- *Regimen A*: Ofloxacin 400 mg PO *bid,* plus metronidazole 500 mg PO *bid* for 14 days
- *Regimen B*: Ceftriaxone 250 mg IM or cefoxitin 2.0 g IM (plus probenecid 1.0 g PO), plus doxycycline 100 mg PO *bid* for 14 days

Supportive Therapy   Promptly remove IUD, if present; bedrest may speed subjective improvement in severe cases; analgesics as needed; advise sexual abstention for at least 2 weeks

Follow-Up   Reexamine at 1- to 3-day intervals until improved; clinical progression at any time or failure to improve within 3–4 days is indication for laparoscopic diagnosis and parenteral therapy; after improvement begins, reexamine weekly until clinically resolved

CONTROL MEASURES

Management of Sex Partners   Examine all partners, even when immediate sexual acquisition of PID seems unlikely (such as IUD-related PID in a monogamous patient); unless sexual acquisition excluded with certainty, treat partners for presumptive gonorrhea and chlamydial infection

Reporting   Report gonococcal or chlamydial infection according to local regulations

Counseling   Counsel patient about sexually transmitted nature of PID and risks for infertility (15–30% for each episode of PID) and ectopic pregnancy; avoid nonspecific terms, such as "infected ovarian cyst," and others that deemphasize the sexually transmitted nature of PID

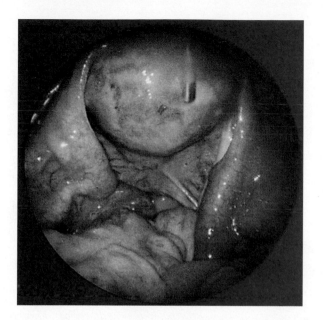

19–1. *Laparoscopic view of pelvic structures in acute PID (not from patient described), showing normal uterus (under probe) anteriorly; left fallopian tube (left side of figure) has slight edema with reddened, agglutinated fimbria; right tube is mildly swollen and erythematous; purulent exudate is seen deep in cul-de-sac. (Courtesy of David E. Soper, M.D.)*

Patient Profile Age 18, grocery clerk

History Increased vaginal discharge for 10 days; mild low abdominal pain and dyspareunia for 4 days, severe pain for 1 day; no fever or chills; monogamous with current boyfriend for 3 months; no past history of STD

Examination Afebrile; bilateral lower quadrant abdominal tenderness, without rebound; edematous cervical ectopy and mucopurulent cervical exudate; homogeneous white vaginal fluid; moderate cervical motion, fundal and adnexal tenderness bilaterally; left adnexal fullness, without overt mass

Differential Diagnosis Pelvic inflammatory disease, ectopic pregnancy, endometriosis, appendicitis, urinary tract infection, colitis

Laboratory Findings of BV and MPC by microscopy, pH, and amine odor test; WBC 8,600 per mm^3 with normal differential; ESR 35 mm/h; endocervical culture positive for *C. trachomatis,* negative for *N. gonorrhoeae;* VDRL and HIV serology negative

Diagnosis Pelvic inflammatory disease due to *C. trachomatis*

Treatment Ofloxacin 400 mg PO *bid* plus metronidazole 500 mg PO *bid* for 14 days

Partner Management Advised to refer partner for examination and treatment; partner found to have asymptomatic urethral chlamydial infection; treated with azithromycin 1.0 g PO, single dose

Follow-Up Reexamined 2 days later; pain improved, with reduced adnexal tenderness; counseled regarding STD prevention and risks of infertility and ectopic pregnancy; scheduled to be retested for *C. trachomatis* 3 months later (rescreening; see Chap. 2)

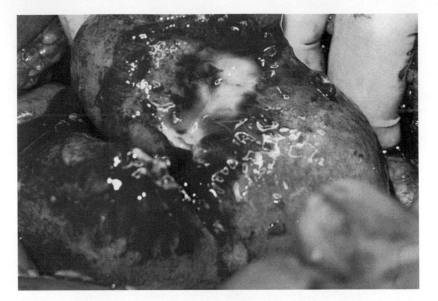

19–2. *Tubo-ovarian abscess in severe PID (not in patient described): lower half of figure is bilobed pyosalpinx/abscess, which was adherent to uterine fundus (above center); purulent exudate is present at junction of uterus and pyosalpinx. (Courtesy of David E. Soper, M.D., reprinted with permission from DE Soper,* Am J Obstet Gynecol *164:1370, 1991.*

Patient Profile   Age 32, married schoolteacher

History   Intermittent, mild, low abdominal pain and vaginal discharge since IUD inserted 4 months earlier; severe abdominal pain, fever, chills, nausea, and vomiting for 1 day; denied extramarital sex partners

Examination   Temperature 39.2°C orally; bilateral lower quadrant direct and rebound abdominal tenderness; profuse mucopurulent cervical discharge; marked bilateral pelvic tenderness, with suggestion of right adnexal mass (examination compromised by tenderness and guarding)

Differential Diagnosis   Pelvic inflammatory disease, appendicitis, ectopic pregnancy, severe endometriosis

Laboratory   Stat pelvic ultrasound showed 6- by 38-cm fluid-filled mass with internal echoes, plus small effusion in cul-de-sac; WBC 14,700 per mm^3 with 80% PMNs; ESR 50 mm/h; cervical Gram stain and vaginal saline mount showed many PMNs and clue cells, without trichomonads or yeasts; vaginal pH 5.0, KOH amine odor positive; negative cultures for *N. gonorrhoeae* and *C. trachomatis*; 2 blood cultures sent (later reported negative); VDRL and HIV serology negative

Diagnosis   IUD-related PID with tubo-ovarian abscess

Treatment   Patient hospitalized; IUD removed; treated with IV clindamycin and gentamicin

Partner Management   Husband referred for examination; denied other sex partners, examination normal; negative urine LCR tests for *C. trachomatis* and *N. gonorrhoeae*; not treated

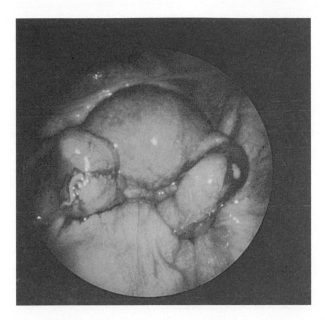

19-3. *Bilateral pyosalpinx in severe PID; pus is seen exuding from left tube (left side of figure) after needle aspiration for culture. (Courtesy of David E. Soper, M.D.; reprinted with permission from DE Soper,* Am J Obstet Gynecol *164:1370, 1991.)*

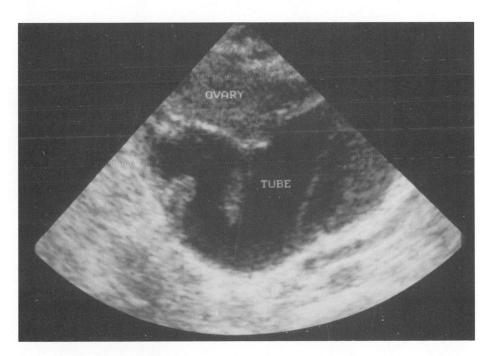

19-4. *Pelvic ultrasound examination in acute PID with pyosalpinx. (Courtesy of Faye Laing, M.D.)*

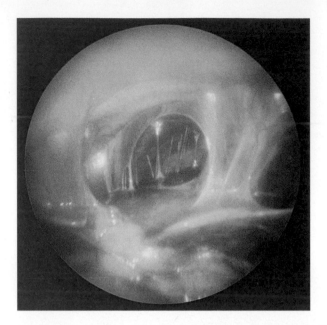

19–5. *Adhesions between liver (below) and parietal peritoneum in a woman with acute perihepatitis (Fitz-Hugh–Curtis syndrome) due to* C. trachomatis. *(Courtesy of David E. Soper, M.D.)*

ADDITIONAL READING

Cohen CR, Brunham RC: Pathogenesis of chlamydia-induced pelvic inflammatory disease. *Sex Transm Infect* 75:21–24, 1999. *An up-to-date review of the immunopathology of PID and the relationship of pathogenesis to prevention and treatment.*

Merchant JS et al: Douching: a problem for adolescent girls and young women. *Arch Pediatr Adolesc Med* 153:834–837, 1999. *Comprehensive review and meta-analysis of the literature associating vaginal douching with PID and ectopic pregnancy.*

Walker CK et al: Anaerobes in pelvic inflammatory disease: implications for the Centers for Disease Control and Prevention's guidelines for treatment of sexually transmitted diseases. *Clin Infect Dis* 28 (Suppl 1):S29–S36, 1999. *Review of therapy of PID and the controversies regarding anaerobic bacteria in its pathogenesis; background paper for CDC's 1998 STD treatment guidelines.*

Weström L, Eschenbach DE: Pelvic inflammatory disease, in *Sexually Transmitted Diseases,* 3rd ed, KK Holmes et al (eds). New York, McGraw-Hill, 1999, Chap 58. *A comprehensive review by two premier experts on PID.*

Chapter 20
PROCTITIS, COLITIS, AND ENTERITIS

Sexually acquired proctitis can be caused by *Neisseria gonorrhoeae, Chlamydia trachomatis,* herpes simplex virus (HSV), and *Treponema pallidum,* which are acquired by direct rectal exposure or, in women, anal exposure to infected cervicovaginal secretions. Enteritis, or small intestinal infection, is sexually transmitted through practices that foster oral exposure to feces. The most common recognized sexually transmitted enteritis is giardiasis, but cryptosporidiosis, microsporidiosis, isosporiasis, and other enteric infections undoubtedly can be transmitted by this mechanism. Sexually acquired colitis and proctocolitis result either from fecal–oral contamination (e.g., amebiasis, shigellosis) or rectal inoculation (e.g., lymphogranuloma venereum, LGV). *Campylobacter* infection and salmonellosis, acquired orally, may result in enteritis, colitis, or both syndrome (enterocolitis). All sexually active persons are susceptible to these infections, but the practices conducive to their transmission are most frequent among MSM. Most cases of sexually transmitted enteritis, colitis, and proctocolitis are clinically indistinguishable from nonsexually acquired syndromes, such as inflammatory bowel disease and foodborne or waterborne infections.

EPIDEMIOLOGY

Incidence and Prevalence   Highly variable, depending on sexual practices; reliable statistics not available

Transmission   Receptive anal intercourse; fecal–oral contamination (e.g., analingus and contaminated hands or sex toys); some rectal infections in women (e.g., gonorrhea) and acquired through contiguous spread of cervicovaginal infections

Age   No specific predilection, except for influence of age on sexual behavior

Sex and Sexual Orientation   Most common in MSM; probably least common in exclusively heterosexual men

Other Risk Factors   Persons with HIV infection may be at increased risk of sexually acquired opportunistic gastrointestinal infections (e.g., cryptosporidiosis)

HISTORY

Incubation Period   Variable, depending on specific infection

Symptoms

- *Proctitis*: Anal pain, tenesmus, constipation, bleeding; anal or perianal ulcers or vesiculo-

pustular lesions (herpes, syphilis); fever or systemic symptoms suggest primary herpes or LGV; sacral neuropathy (e.g., bladder paralysis) suggests primary herpes
- *Colitis*: Diarrhea, sometimes bloody; abdominal cramps; often fever or other systemic symptoms
- *Enteritis*: Diarrhea, usually without cramping; variable nausea, vomiting, anorexia, bloating, flatulence, weight loss, fever
- *Proctocolitis, enterocolitis*: Simultaneous symptoms of component syndromes

Epidemiologic History   History of exposure; high-risk sexual practices

PHYSICAL EXAMINATION

Proctitis   Anoscopy or sigmoidoscopy demonstrates various combinations of mucosal erythema, extending no higher than 10 cm above anus; purulent exudate, sometimes emanating from anal crypts; mucosal ulcers or petechiae; sometimes bleeding induced by swabbing rectal mucosa ("wipe test"); sometimes ulcers or vesiculopustules of anal canal or perianally

Colitis and Proctocolitis   Abdominal tenderness, usually maximum in left lower quadrant; often fever; sigmoidoscopy or colonoscopy with inflammation >10 cm beyond anus; proctocolitis causes clinical signs and mucosal changes consistent with both proctitis and colitis

Enteritis and Enterocolitis   Often no physical findings; sometimes abdominal tenderness or enhanced bowel sounds

DIFFERENTIAL AND LABORATORY DIAGNOSIS

Proctitis   Most MSM with acute proctitis have gonorrhea, chlamydial infection, herpes, or primary or secondary syphilis; differential diagnosis probably similar in sexually active women, but poorly studied; anoscopy for visual inspection and clinical specimens, including Gram-stained smear, culture or DNA amplification tests for *N. gonorrhoeae* and *C. trachomatis,* culture for HSV; VDRL; type-specific HSV serology; darkfield examination; rectal biopsy sometimes required

Colitis and Proctocolitis   Usual causes are *C. trachomatis* (especially LGV strains), *Campylobacter jejuni, Shigella* sp., *Salmonella* sp., and *Entamoeba histolytica;* all may be clinically indistinguishable from ulcerative colitis or Crohn's disease; examine by sigmoidoscopy or colonoscopy; culture for *N. gonorrhoeae, C. trachomatis,* and HSV; stool for leukocytes, culture, and ova and parasite examination; chlamydia/LGV serology if LGV suspected; biopsy sometimes helpful, but LGV is histologically indistinguishable from Crohn's disease

Enteritis and Enterocolitis   Broad differential diagnosis, including *Campylobacter* and *Salmonella*; in MSM, *Giardia lamblia* is most common cause of enteritis without colitis; in HIV-infected and other immunocompromised persons, consider *Cryptosporidium, Isospora, Cyclospora,* microsporidia, CMV, and *Mycobacterium avium* complex; examine stool for leukocytes; stool culture; ova and parasite examination; consider "string test" of duodenal secretions for *G. lamblia*; colonoscopy, upper gastrointestinal endoscopy, and mucosal biopsy often indicated

TREATMENT

Proctitis and Proctocolitis   Treat according to specific cause (see Chaps. 2–4, 7); consider presumptive therapy on basis of clinical findings, pending test results (e.g., benzathine penicillin plus valacyclovir for ulcerative proctitis suggestive of syphilis or herpes, cefixime plus doxycycline if ulcers absent); treat LGV proctocolitis with doxycycline 100 mg PO *bid* for 3 weeks (see Chap. 2)

Colitis and Enterocolitis

AMEBIASIS   For overt colitis or other invasive amebiasis, use metronidazole 750 mg PO *tid* for 10 days, followed by iodoquinol 650 mg PO *tid* for 3 weeks; for asymptomatic carriage, iodoquinol 650 mg PO *tid* for 3 weeks, or paromomycin 10 mg/kg body weight *tid* plus diloxanide furoate 500 mg PO *tid* for 3 weeks

SALMONELLOSIS   Most cases resolve promptly without antimicrobial therapy; for severe infection requiring treatment, use ciprofloxacin 500 mg PO *bid* (or other fluoroquinolone in equivalent dosage) for 7 days, pending susceptibility tests

SHIGELLOSIS   Most cases do not require specific therapy; for severe infection requiring treatment, use ciprofloxacin 500 mg PO *bid* (or other fluoroquinolone in equivalent dosage) for 7 days, pending susceptibility tests

CAMPYLOBACTER INFECTION   Mild cases usually require no treatment; for severe infections, use azithromycin 500 mg PO daily for 3 days, or erythromycin 500 mg PO *qid* for 7 days

Enteritis

GIARDIASIS   Metronidazole 250–500 mg PO *tid* for 7 days; paromomycin 500 mg PO *tid* for 7–10 days; or furazolidone 100 mg PO *qid* for 7–10 days

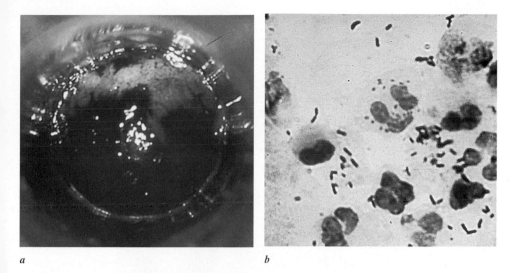

a   b

20–1.   a. *Gonococcal proctitis: anoscopic view of purulent exudate and mucosal bleeding (positive "wipe test").* b. *Gram-stained smear of rectal exudate, showing a single PMN with ICGND. (Part* b *reprinted with permission from KK Holmes et al (eds),* Sexually Transmitted Diseases, *3d ed. New York, McGraw-Hill, 1999.)*

Patient Profile   Age 34, unemployed, methamphetamine-addicted gay man

History   Anal discharge, pruritus, and blood in stools for 3 days; no diarrhea, cramps, fever, or systemic symptoms; frequent unprotected sex with anonymous partners

Examination   Genitals normal; anus normal; anoscopy showed purulent exudate and mucosal fri ability with spontaneous bleeding, enhanced by swabbing (positive "wipe test")

Differential Diagnosis   Gonorrhea, herpes, chlamydial infection (including LGV), syphilis

Laboratory   Gram stain of rectal exudate showed for PMNs, rare cells with ICGND; rectal culture for *N. gonorrhoeae* (positive); rectal cultures for *C. trachomatis* and HSV (both negative); darkfield examination, stat RPR, VDRL, HIV serology (all negative)

Diagnosis   Gonococcal proctitis

Treatment   Cefixime 400 mg PO, single dose, plus doxycycline 100 mg PO *bid* for 7 days

Partner Management   Patient was unable to identify sex partners

Comment   Rectal Gram stain permitted presumptive diagnosis and immediate specific therapy for gonorrhea; symptoms resolved over next 2 days; patient returned 2 weeks later with sore throat, fever, and skin rash, and was diagnosed with primary HIV infection

---

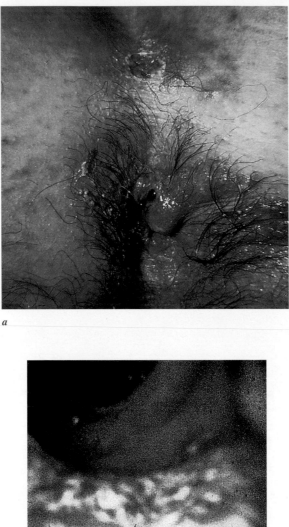

a

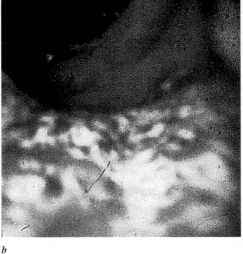

b

20–2. *Acute proctitis due to primary herpes in a gay man who presented with 5 days of severe perianal pain, tenesmus, difficulty urinating, fever, and headache.* a. *Perianal ulcer, anal edema, and purulent anal discharge.* b. *Mucosal ulcers and exudate viewed by fiberoptic sigmoidoscopy. (Part b courtesy of Christina M. Surawicz, M.D.)*

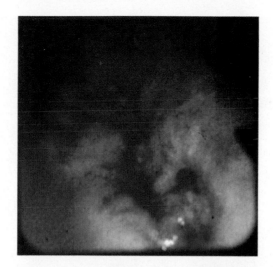

20–3. *Proctitis due to* Chlamydia trachomatis *(non–LGV strain), showing mucosal erythema and edema, viewed by fiberoptic sigmoidoscopy. (Courtesy of Thomas Quinn, M.D.)*

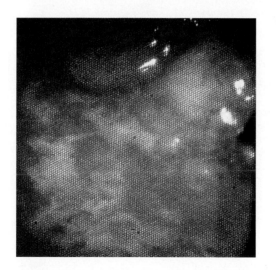

20–4. *Gonococcal proctitis: purulent rectal exudate viewed by fiberoptic sigmoidoscopy. (Courtesy of Christina M. Surawicz, M.D.)*

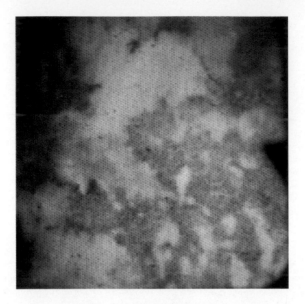

20–5. *Amebic proctocolitis: rectal mucosal ulcerations, exudate, and petechiae due to amebic proctocolitis, viewed by fiberoptic sigmoidoscopy. Note similarity to herpetic and gonococcal proctitis (Figs. 20–2, 20–4). (Courtesy of Thomas Quinn, M.D.)*

ADDITIONAL READING

Rompalo AM: Diagnosis and treatment of sexually acquired proctitis and proctocolitis: an update. *Clin Infect Dis* 28 (Suppl 1):S84–S90, 1999. *A comprehensive, well-written review by one of the prominent investigators in the field.*

Verley JR, Quinn TC: Sexually transmitted intestinal syndromes, in *Sexually Transmitted Diseases,* 3ed, KK Holmes et al (eds). New York, McGraw-Hill, 1999, Chap 69. *A comprehensive review in the main textbook on sexually transmitted diseases.*

Chapter 21
NONSEXUALLY TRANSMITTED GENITAL DERMATOSES

Many dermatologic conditions can affect the genitals, and some anatomic variants occasionally are confused with abnormal conditions by patients or their health care providers. Not surprisingly, sexually active persons with genital dermatoses often present to providers with concerns about STD. Entire textbooks have been written on the topic of genital dermatology, and it is beyond the scope of this book to provide a comprehensive overview. Examples of a few conditions are presented, with emphasis on those that are especially likely to affect younger persons or that are easily confused with STDs.

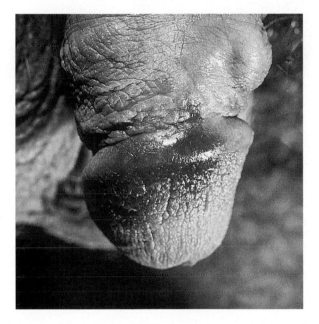

21–1. *Fixed drug eruption of the penis. The patient had just finished a 7-day course of tetracycline HCl for NGU and complained of 3 days of pain "like a burn."*

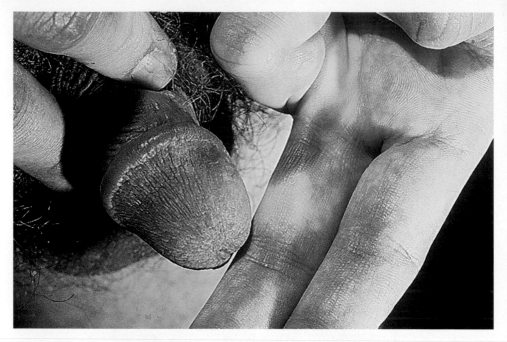

21–2. *Fixed drug eruption, with sharply demarcated erythematous lesions of the glans penis and finger web in a patient treated with doxycycline for chlamydial infection.*

Comment   Fixed drug eruptions typically (Figs. 21–1 and 21–2) are localized reactions to systemic allergens that often involve the genitals, sometimes leading to confusion with STDs. Recurrent episodes typically involve the identical areas as the first episode. In addition to the tetracyclines, fixed drug eruptions can be caused by sulfonamides, metronidazole, phenytoin, phenolphthalein, and others. The lesion typically resembles a burn, with initial pain and erythema followed by superficial sloughing. The reaction typically begins 7–10 days after initiating the offending drug, but the onset may be faster with subsequent exposures. Healing occurs without scarring, although hyperpigmentation may persist. Aside from discontinuing the offending drug, no specific treatment is available.

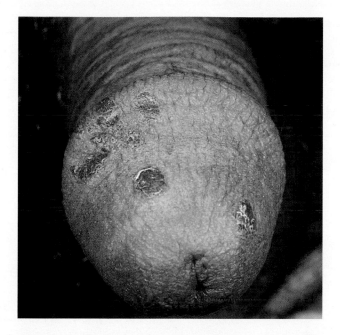

21–3. *Psoriasis of the penis. Having begun a new sexual relationship 2 weeks previously, the patient suspected STD; he also had a previously unrecognized patch of typical psoriasis of the scalp.*

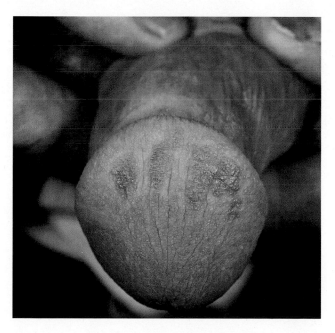

21–4. *Psoriasis of the penis.*

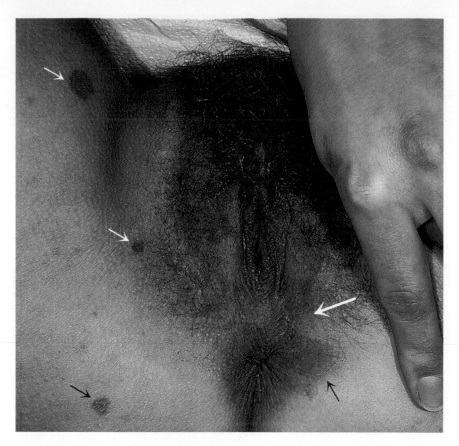

21–5. *Psoriasis; several psoriatic plaques (black arrows) in a woman with recurrent genital herpes (white arrow).*

Comment   Psoriasis often involves the genitals and can mimic secondary syphilis (Fig. 4–13), scabies (Fig. 13–2), and keratoderma blennorrhagica of Reiter's syndrome. Most patients have psoriasis of other sites, but genital lesions may be the first or only manifestations. Sometimes biopsy is necessary for diagnosis.

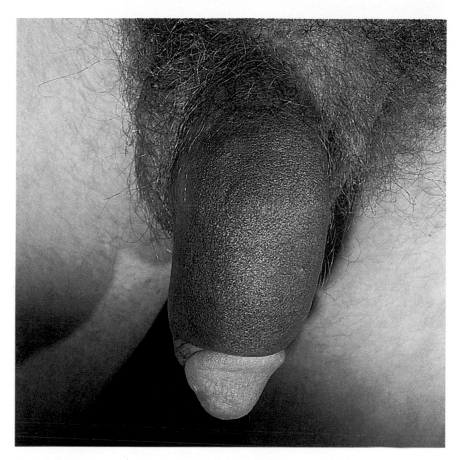

21–6. *Penile hemorrhage due to corpus cavernosum fracture. The patient presented to an STD clinic 1 hour after sudden onset of extreme pain and swelling that began when his sex partner rolled onto his erect penis.*

Comment "Penile fracture" is rupture of a corpus cavernosum, a rare event that typically results from forcible flexion of the penis when erect. Surgery is required to repair the capsule of the ruptured corpus to preserve nondeformed erections in the future.

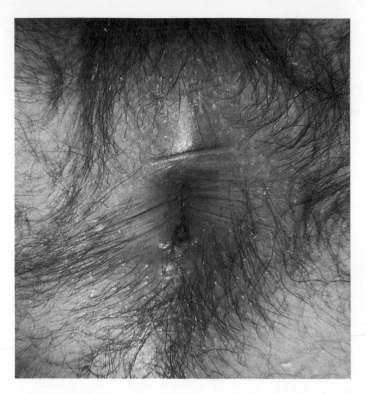

21–7. *Anal fissure in a man presenting with anal pain and occasional bleeding for 1 week. (Courtesy of Steven J. Medwell, M.D.)*

Comment   Anal fissures are common in all populations, but may be particularly frequent in MSM and women who participate in receptive anal intercourse. Note similarity to anal lesions of primary syphilis (Fig. 4–10) and herpes (Fig. 7–16). Sexually active persons who present with anal fissures should be asked about receptive anal sex; many should be evaluated for STD.

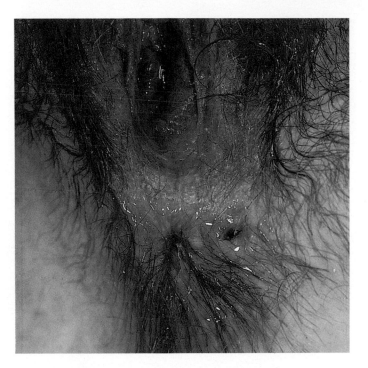

21–8. *Chronic rectal fistula with gonorrhea.*

Comment   This patient presented to an STD clinic with 1 week of drainage from a "sore" next to her anus, as well as occasional uncontrolled fecal leakage and flatus from the same area for several months. About 1 year earlier she had painful swelling near the anus that resolved when a large "boil" drained spontaneously. *Neisseria gonorrhoeae* was isolated from her cervix, anal canal, and the fistula tract.

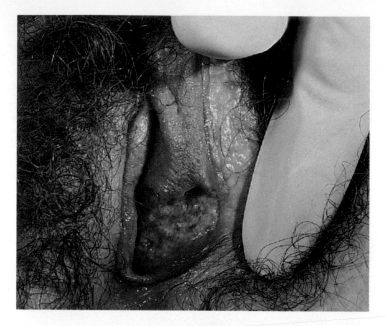

21–9.   *Genital ulcer due to Behçet's syndrome in a 23-year-old woman born in Turkey; the patient also had several years of deeply erosive oral aphthous ulcers.*

Comment   Behçet's syndrome is a rare, often serious condition of probable autoimmune origin, usually in persons of Mediterranean ancestry. It is manifested by recurrent, often deeply erosive, oral and genital ulcers and often by conjunctivitis or uveitis. Complications include arthritis, erythema nodosum, cranial neuropathies, and arteritis that can result in blindness from retinal infarction, meningoencephalitis, stroke, and psychosis. Colchicine, corticosteroids, chlorambucil, and other cytotoxic drugs are used for treatment, with variable efficacy.

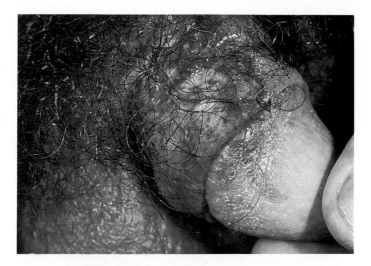

21–10. *Staphylococcal pyoderma of the penis in a patient with scabies.*

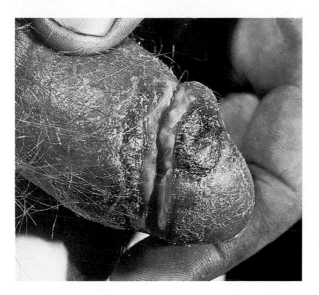

21–11. *Penile pyoderma with necrotizing cellulitis in a man with secondary syphilis;* Staphylococcus aureus *and β-hemolytic* Streptococcus pyogenes *were isolated. This is the same patient whose skin rash due to secondary syphilis is shown in Fig. 4–19; he gave a history of a painless ulcer at the corona of the penis for the preceding 6 weeks.*

Comment Pyoderma of the penis usually results from secondary infection of a preexisting lesion. Scabies is a common predisposing factor. For unknown reasons, secondary infection of herpetic lesions or syphilitic chancres is uncommon, although a chancre probably was the initial lesion in the patient in Figure 21–11. Hospitalization may be required for severe cases to preserve penile viability; the patient in Figure 21–11 responded to intravenous antibiotics, except that part of the glans (under the black eschar) sloughed.

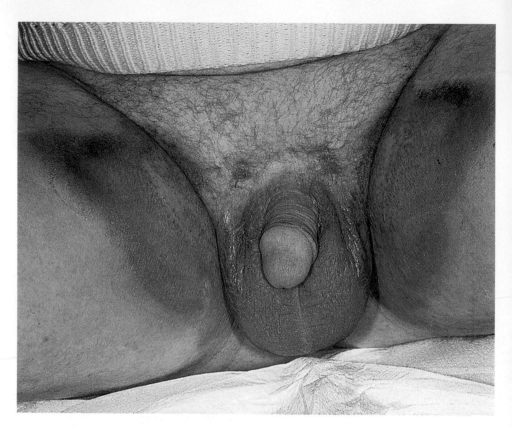

21–12. *Erythrasma.*

Comment   Erythrasma is a superficial cutaneous infection, typically of the genitals, upper thighs, and crural folds, caused by *Corynebacterium minutissimum*. Most cases are less extensive than illustrated in Fig. 21–12. Bright coral-red fluorescence is seen under ultraviolet light (Wood's lamp). Chronic cases typically present with a copper-colored, red-brown rash with a raised border and often with fine scale. Erythrasma can be confused with tinea cruris (Fig. 21–13); the distinction is important because the treatments are different. The treatment is oral erythromycin; clarithromycin also is effective.

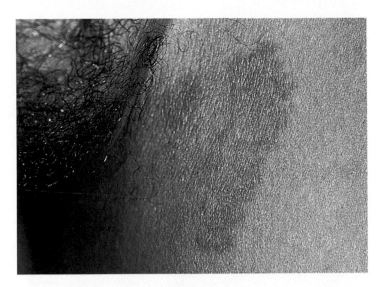

21–13.   *Tinea cruris in a woman. (Courtesy of Philip Kirby, M.D.)*

Comment   Tinea cruris is most common in men ("jock itch") but is not rare in women. It is caused by dermatophyte fungi, including *Trichophyton, Epidermophyton,* and *Microsporum* species, and tinea pedis (athlete's foot) often is present. Tinea cruris is characterized by an erythematous, papular, sometimes erosive dermatitis of the crural folds, inner thighs, or scrotum, with accentuated erythema and fine scale at the sharply demarcated border. The clinical diagnosis usually is reliable, but can be confirmed by scraping the advancing border and examining microscopically for fungal elements after digestion with 10% KOH. Topical imidazole creams (e.g., miconazole) are effective.

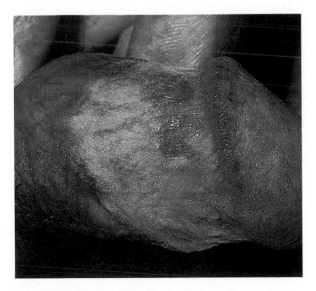

21–14.   *Vitiligo of the penis. (Courtesy of Philip Kirby, M.D.)*

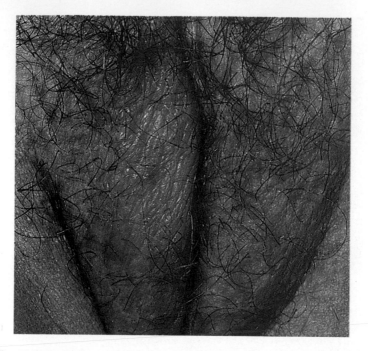

21–15. *Lichen simplex chronicus of the vulva, with an ulcer caused by excoriation.*

Comment   Lichen simplex chronicus (Fig. 21–15) usually presents as a solitary plaque with thickening of the skin and accentuated markings (lichenification), erythema, and sometimes excoriation reflecting intense pruritus. Vulvar or scrotal involvement are typical; the condition is more common in women than men. The underlying cause is unknown, but most of the clinical manifestations result from habitual scratching (which may be unconscious) and lesions are most common on the side of the dominant hand. Topical steroids and instruction to avoid scratching often are effective; dressings may be necessary to prevent unconscious scratching during sleep.

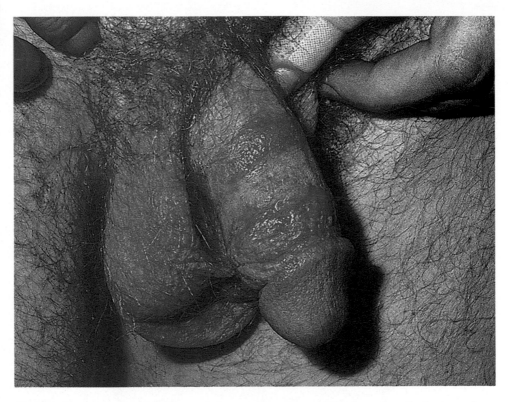

21–16. *Contact dermatitis of the penis in a patient who was allergic to the adhesive tape of a bandage used to cover an episode of recurrent genital herpes; healing herpetic lesions are visible between the patches of acute dermatitis.*

Comment In its fully developed form, allergic contact dermatitis is characterized by vesicles or a denuded, weeping skin surface. History of exposure to potential irritants or allergens often is present. Removal of the inciting agent usually results in prompt resolution, although topical steroids may speed improvement.

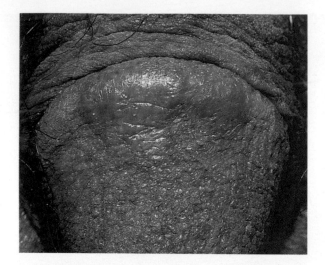

21–17. *Lichen planus of the penis. (Courtesy of Karl R. Beutner, M.D., Ph.D.)*

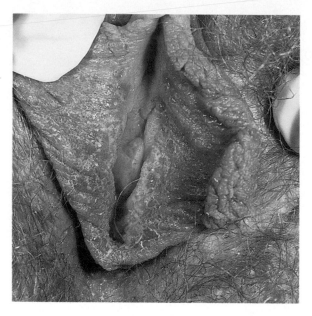

21–18. *Lichen planus of the vaginal introitus, with faintly violaceous, serpiginous striations. Secondary lichenification of the labia minora also is present.*

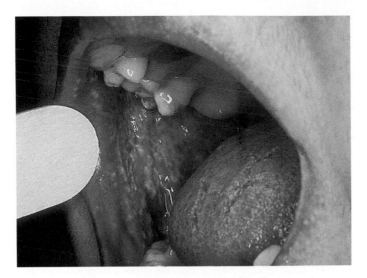

21–19. *Lichen planus of the oral mucosa.*

Comment   Lichen planus is one of the more common genital dermatoses and is seen frequently in patients at risk for STD. The condition typically causes flat-topped papules with shiny surfaces, often with a violaceous hue. Most lesions itch, but some are nonpruritic. Oral or genital mucosal lesions often are present, with lacy, serpiginous striae; when the lateral aspect of the tongue is involved, lichen planus can mimic HIV-related hairy leukoplakia. The cause is unknown; most cases respond to topical corticosteroids.

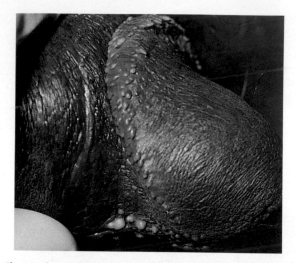

21–20. *Pearly penile papules and Tyson's glands. There are numerous pearly penile papules along the corona of the glans penis; the larger white papules on the ventral surface below the glans are Tyson's glands. (Courtesy of Philip Kirby, M.D.)*

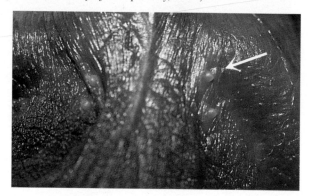

21–21. *Four Tyson's glands, one of which is denoted by a white arrow. (Courtesy of Karl R. Beutner, M.D., Ph.D.)*

Comment   Pearly penile papules are normal anatomic variants that appear as small (usually 0.5–1 mm) shiny papules of the penile corona; prominent papules may have a filiform morphology. They are present in 10–20% of men, regardless of race or skin color, and are more common in circumcised than uncircumcised men. Tyson's glands are prominent, specialized sebaceous glands, symmetrically located on the ventral aspect of the penis immediately proximal to the glans; one, two, or sometimes three pairs may be present. Some affected men become concerned after first noticing pearly penile papules or Tyson's glands (e.g., after observing other men without them), and naive clinicians may confuse them with genital warts, molluscum contagiosum, or other lesions.

ADDITIONAL READING

Fitzpatrick TB et al: *Color Atlas and Synopsis of Clinical Dermatology,* 4th ed. New York, McGraw-Hill, 2001. *A comprehensive (1072 pages), extensively illustrated review of dermatologic conditions, with format and approach similar to this book.*
Lynch PJ, Edwards MD: *Genital Dermatology.* New York, Churchill Livingstone, 1994. *A well-illustrated, brief text of dermatoses that commonly affect the genitals.*

Appendix
MEDICAL AND SEXUAL HISTORY, PHYSICAL EXAMINATION, AND LABORATORY EVALUATION OF STD PATIENTS

This outline is derived from the clinical record of the Public Health—Seattle & King County STD Clinic.* All elements can be expressed in check-off format or with numerical entries. In the author's clinic, separate male and female records are printed on two sides of a single page, with sufficient space for expanded written findings.

MEDICAL HISTORY

Reason(s) for Visit
Symptoms
STD screen (asymptomatic)
HIV test
Positive STD test (specify)
Referral (specify source)
STD exposure (specify disease)

Symptoms and Duration

MALES
Urethral symptoms (discharge, dysuria, other)
Genital lesion or rash
Nongenital rash
Anorectal symptoms
Testicular symptoms
Oropharyngeal symptoms
Other (specify)

FEMALES
Vulvovaginal symptoms (discharge, odor, pruritus)
Dysuria (specify external or internal)
Urinary urgency or frequency
Genital lesion or rash
Abdominal or pelvic pain or dyspareunia
Abnormal vaginal bleeding
Nongenital rash
Anorectal symptoms
Oropharyngeal symptoms
Other (specify)

Other Medical History
Drug allergies
Antibiotics and antiviral drugs in past month

HIV RISK ASSESSMENT

HIV Status
Positive
  Receiving HIV health care?
  On antiretroviral therapy?
  Any HIV-negative needle-sharing or sex partners (or partners of unknown HIV status) in past 12 months?
Negative
Never tested
Date of last test

Risk Assessment (past year, ever, most recent)
Sex with a gay or bisexual man
Sex with an injection drug user (IDU)
Sex with HIV-infected person
Injection drug use
Exchange of drugs or money for sex
Multiple (e.g., ≥4) opposite sex partners in past year
Other risk (specify)
None of the above

SEXUAL HISTORY AND PRACTICES

Partnerships
Gender of sex partners in past year (male, female, both)
Sexual exposures (elicited separately for opposite-sex and same-sex partners)
  Number of partners, past 2 months and 12 months
  Days since last sex with regular sex partner
  Days since first sex with a new partner

Anatomic sites exposed in past 2 months (penis, vagina, rectum, mouth/throat)
Condom use during most recent penile-insertive sex
For men who have sex with men:
Anonymous (i.e., unidentifiable) partners in past 2 months
Frequency of condom use in past 2 months (never, sometimes, usually, always; asked separately for anal insertive and anal receptive intercourse)

Past STD (yes/no and most recent episode)
Chlamydia
NGU (men only)
Trichomoniasis (women only)
BV (women only)
PID (women only)
Gonorrhea
Syphilis
Genital herpes
Genital warts

OBSTETRIC AND GYNECOLOGIC HISTORY (WOMEN)

Date of last normal menstrual period
Parity
Most recent cervical cytology (date, result)
Douching in past year (yes/no)
Contraceptive method(s) in past 2 months

PHYSICAL EXAMINATION

Males

Circumcision status
Urethral discharge, amount and character (clear, mucopurulent, purulent)
Genital lesions (description, location, number, size)
Scrotal/testicular palpation
Lymphadenopathy
Inguinal
Other
Anorectal examination if symptomatic or history of anal exposure
Visual inspection of anus, perineum
Anoscopy (selected patients)
Skin (examine all exposed skin surfaces)
Oropharyngeal inspection

Females

Vulva and introitus; describe and enumerate lesions
Vagina and vaginal secretions
Amount: None, small, moderate, large
Color and character (white, yellow, brown, bloody; floccular, homogenous, adherent plaques)
Cervix
Lesions
Ectopy (extent, edema)
Swab-induced endocervical bleeding
Exudate (amount, color, character)
Bimanual pelvic examination
Cervical motion tenderness
Uterine fundus (size, form, tenderness)
Adnexal tenderness
Adnexal or other pelvic mass
Lymphadenopathy
Inguinal
Other
Anorectal examination
Visual inspection of anus, perineum
Anoscopy (selected patients)
Skin (examine all exposed skin surfaces)
Oropharyngeal inspection

LABORATORY[†]

Immediate Microscopy and Other Rapid Tests

Gram-stained smear (urethra, cervix, rectum, vaginal fluid)
Wet-mount microscopy (saline and 10% KOH)
Vaginal fluid pH
Vaginal fluid amine odor (KOH "sniff") test
Darkfield microscopy
Rapid plasma reagin (or other rapid syphilis serology)
Leukocyte esterase
Urinalysis (dipstick, microscopy)
Microscopy of skin scrapings for scabies
Rapid pregnancy testing

Microbiologic and Virologic Tests

Neisseria gonorrhoeae
Chlamydia trachomatis
Herpes simplex virus

[†]The tests listed should be readily available in STD clinics and other settings frequently attended by patients with STD or at risk. However, even STD clinics may find it impractical to have routine testing available for rare conditions (e.g., tests for *Haemophilus ducreyi* in settings where chancroid is absent). The selection of tests for routine screening or diagnosis varies with patients' symptoms, exposure history, epidemiologic circumstances, the local prevalence and incidence of various STDs, and specific assays available in local or regional laboratories. See Chap. 1 for recommendations for routine STD assessment in most primary care settings.

Haemophilus ducreyi
Trichomonas vaginalis
Candida species
Urine culture for standard uropathogens

Serological Tests
Syphilis serology (reaginic and confirmatory assays)
HIV serology; other diagnostic tests in selected settings (HIV viral load, CD4 lymphocyte assay)
HSV type-specific serological test
Viral hepatitis serology (HAV, HBV; HCV optional)

Other
Cervical cytology (Pap smear)

INDEX

ISBN 0-07-026033-8 NB2I

90000

9 780070 260337

HANDSFIELD/COLOR ATLAS
SYNOPSIS STDS